Diagnosis and Management of Neck Masses

Editor

DAVID E. WEBB

ATLAS OF THE ORAL AND MAXILLOFACIAL SURGERY CLINICS OF NORTH AMERICA

www.oralmaxsurgeryatlas.theclinics.com

Consulting Editor
RICHARD H. HAUG

March 2015 • Volume 23 • Number 1

ELSEVIER

1600 John F. Kennedy Boulevard • Suite 1800 • Philadelphia, Pennsylvania, 19103-2899
http://www.oralmaxsurgeryatlas.theclinics.com

ATLAS OF THE ORAL AND MAXILLOFACIAL SURGERY CLINICS OF NORTH AMERICA Volume 23, Number 1
March 2015 ISSN 1061-3315 ISBN-13: 978-0-323-35650-3

Editor: John Vassallo; j.vassallo@elsevier.com
Developmental Editor: Colleen Viola

Reprints. For copies of 100 or more of articles in this publication, please contact the Commercial Reprints Department, Elsevier Inc., 360 Park Avenue South, New York, NY 10010-1710. Tel.: 212-633-3874; Fax: 212-633-3820; E-mail: reprints@elsevier.com.

Atlas of the Oral and Maxillofacial Surgery Clinics of North America (ISSN 1061-3315) is published biannually by Elsevier, 360 Park Avenue South, New York, NY 10010-1710. Months of issue are March and September. Periodicals postage paid at New York, NY and additional mailing offices. Subscription prices are $455.00 for international individual, $370.00 for US individual and Canadian individual; $220.00 for international student and Canadian student, $180.00 for US student; $451.00 for international institution and Canadian institution, $366.00 for US institution. Foreign air speed delivery is included in all *Clinics* subscription prices. All prices are subject to change without notice. POSTMASTER: Send address changes to *Atlas of the Oral and Maxillofacial Surgery Clinics of North America*, Health Sciences Division, Subscription Customer Service, 3251 Riverport Lane, Maryland Heights, MO 63043. Tel: 1-800-654-2452 (U.S. and Canada); 314-447-8871 (outside U.S. and Canada). Fax: 314-417-8029. E-mail: journalscustomerservice-usa@elsevier.com (for print support); journalsonline support-usa@elsevier.com (for online support).

Atlas of the Oral and Maxillofacial Surgery Clinics of North America is covered in MEDLINE/PubMed (Index Medicus).

Contributors

CONSULTING EDITOR

RICHARD H. HAUG, DDS
Professor and Chief, Oral Maxillofacial Surgery, Carolinas
Medical Center, Charlotte, North Carolina

EDITOR

MAJ DAVID E. WEBB, DDS, USAF, DC
Attending Oral and Maxillofacial/Head and Neck Surgeon,
Department of Oral and Maxillofacial Surgery, David Grant
USAF Medical Center, Travis AFB, California

AUTHORS

JASON N. BERMAN, MD, FRCPC, FAAP
MSC Clinician Scientist in Pediatric Oncology, Cancer
Care Nova Scotia Peggy Davison Clinician Scientist,
Director, Clinician Investigator Program and Clinician
Scientist Graduate Program; Associate Professor, Division
of Hematology/Oncology; Departments of Pediatrics,
Microbiology and Immunology, and Pathology, IWK
Health Centre, Dalhousie University, Halifax, Nova Scotia,
Canada

PETER A. BRENNAN, MD, FRCS, FRCSI, FDS
Consultant in Oral and Maxillofacial Surgery, Department of
Oral and Maxillofacial Surgery, Queen Alexandra Hospital,
Portsmouth, United Kingdom

TUAN G. BUI, MD, DMD, FACS
Affiliate Assistant Professor, Oral and Maxillofacial Surgery,
Oregon Health and Sciences University; Surgeon, Head
and Neck Surgical Institute, Portland, Oregon

ERIC R. CARLSON, DMD, MD, FACS
Professor and Kelly L. Krahwinkel Chairman, Department
of Oral and Maxillofacial Surgery, Director of Oral and
Maxillofacial Surgery Residency Program; Director of
Oral/Head and Neck Oncologic Surgery Fellowship
Program, University of Tennessee Medical Center, The
University of Tennessee Cancer Institute, Knoxville,
Tennessee

WILLIAM J. CURTIS, DMD, MD
Assistant Professor, Department of Oral and Maxillofacial
Surgery, University of Kentucky College of Dentistry,
Lexington, Kentucky

ERIC J. DIERKS, MD, DMD, FACS
Affiliate Professor, Oral and Maxillofacial Surgery, Oregon
Health and Sciences University; Director of Fellowship in
Head and Neck Oncologic and Microvascular Reconstructive
Surgery, Head and Neck Surgical Institute, Portland, Oregon

SEAN P. EDWARDS, DDS, MD
Associate Professor, Department of Oral and Maxillofacial
Surgery, University of Michigan, Ann Arbor, Michigan

MAJ BRENT A. FELDT, USAF, MC
Department of Otolaryngology, David Grant USAF Medical
Center, California

RUI FERNANDES, MD, DMD
Associate Professor of Surgery, University of Florida College
of Medicine-Jacksonville, Jacksonville, Florida

GHALI E. GHALI, DDS, MD, FACS
Professor and Chairman, Department of Oral and
Maxillofacial Surgery, LSU Health Science Center,
Shreveport, Louisiana

LTC DAVID GROVER, MD, USAF, MC
Interventional Radiologist, Department of Radiology, David
Grant USAF Medical Center, Travis AFB, California

JOSHUA E. LUBEK, DDS, MD, FACS
Assistant Professor and Fellowship Director, Oral-Head Neck
Surgery/Microvascular Surgery, Oncology Program,
Greenebaum Cancer Center, University of Maryland,
Baltimore, Maryland

LTC JOSEPH McDERMOTT, MD, USAF, MC
Pathologist, Department of Pathology, David Grant USAF
Medical Center, Travis AFB, California

MARK ALLEN MILLER, MD, DMD
Resident, Oral and Maxillofacial Surgery, University of Florida
College of Medicine-Jacksonville, Jacksonville, Florida

ANTHONY MORLANDT, DDS, MD
Assistant Professor, Oral Oncology and Microvascular
Surgery, Oral and Maxillofacial Surgery, University of
Alabama at Birmingham, Birmingham, Alabama

LAURA A. MURPHY, MD
Resident, Department of Pediatrics, IWK Health Centre,
Dalhousie University, Halifax, Nova Scotia, Canada

OLIVER J. PEARCE, FRCR, MBBS
Specialist Registrar in Radiology, Department of Radiology,
Queen Alexandra Hospital, Portsmouth, United Kingdom

AMRO SHIHABI, DMD, MD
Former Fellow, Oral-Head Neck Surgery/Microvascular
Surgery, Oncology Program, Greenebaum Cancer Center,
University of Maryland, Baltimore, Maryland

RYAN J. SMART, DMD, MD
Fellow, Head and Neck Surgery/Microvascular
Reconstructive Surgery, Department of Oral and Maxillofacial
Surgery, LSU Health Sciences Center, Shreveport, Louisiana

**JOHN N. ST.J BLYTHE, FRCS (OMFS), FDS, RCS
(Eng), FRCS (Eng)**
Specialist Registrar in Oral and Maxillofacial
Surgery, Department of Oral and Maxillofacial Surgery,
Queen Alexandra Hospital, Portsmouth, United
Kingdom

ELIZABETH A. TILLEY, FRCR, FRCP
Consultant Head and Neck Radiologist, Department of
Radiology, Queen Alexandra Hospital, Portsmouth, United
Kingdom

BRENT B. WARD, DDS, MD
Associate Professor and Fellowship Program Director,
Oral/Head and Oncologic and Microvascular
Reconstructive Surgery, Section of Oral and Maxillofacial
Surgery, University of Michigan Hospitals, Ann Arbor,
Michigan

MAJ DAVID E. WEBB, DDS, USAF, DC
Attending Oral and Maxillofacial/Head and Neck Surgeon,
Department of Oral and Maxillofacial Surgery, David Grant
USAF Medical Center, Travis AFB, California

MELVYN S. YEOH, DMD, MD
Assistant Professor and Program Director, Department of
Oral and Maxillofacial Surgery, LSU Health Sciences Center,
Shreveport, Louisiana

Contents

Reconstruction of Cervical Defects   **105**

Tuan G. Bui and Eric J. Dierks

ATLAS OF THE ORAL AND MAXILLOFACIAL SURGERY CLINICS OF NORTH AMERICA

FORTHCOMING ISSUES

September 2015

Adjuncts for Care of the Surgical Patient
Sidney Bourgeois, *Editor*

March 2016

Orthognathic Surgery
Steven M. Sullivan, *Editor*

PREVIOUS ISSUES

September 2014

Syndromes of the Head and Neck
Dean M. DeLuke, *Editor*

March 2014

Contemporary Rhytidectomy
Landon D. McLain, *Editor*

September 2013

Office Procedures for the Oral and Maxillofacial Surgeon
Stuart E. Lieblich, *Editor*

RELATED INTEREST

Oral and Maxillofacial Surgery Clinics of North America, August 2014, Volume 26, Issue 3
Local and Regional Flaps of the Head and Neck
Din Lam and Robert A. Strauss, *Editors*
Available at: www.oralmaxsurgery.theclinics.com

THE CLINICS ARE NOW AVAILABLE ONLINE!

Access your subscription at:
www.theclinics.com

Preface

Diagnosis and Management of Neck Masses

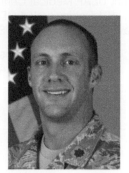

David E. Webb, Maj, USAF, DC
Editor

Mad about surgery

The only people for me are the mad ones, the ones who are mad to live, mad to talk, mad to be saved, desirous of everything at the same time, the ones who never yawn or say a commonplace thing, but burn, burn, burn like fabulous yellow roman candles exploding like spiders across the stars.

—Jack Kerouac, On the Road

Good hands, heads, and hearts

When I was an Oral and Maxillofacial Surgery (OMS) resident, I constantly perseverated about and obsessed over my quest to develop "good hands." I started shaving and brushing my teeth with my nondominant hand, tied silk knots on every imaginable surface, and practiced "palming" a needle driver everywhere I went. Recognizing that outstanding manual dexterity is obviously a must to successfully operate the neck, it is clearly the case that good hands alone don't guarantee good outcomes. In addition to good hands, fellowship training further reinforced the importance of developing a "good head" (ie, cognitive analysis). I learned that our patients are our "books," that each patient is unique and as such requires an individual approach based on guiding principles, and that the answer to every question begins with "It depends—." Feeling well equipped as a new attending, I was surprised to discover that I still lacked a critical component of care—a truly caring

heart. The powerful combination of good hands, heads, and hearts results in surgeons who are truly mad about surgery and whose results are never commonplace, but "burn, burn, burn like fabulous yellow roman candles exploding like spiders across the stars" (*On The Road*). Let us be mad about surgery!

Exciting times

These are exciting times for Oral and Maxillofacial Surgeons. OMS Head and Neck fellowship opportunities have increased over 150% in the last decade (with more on the horizon). Also, an estimated 40% of current OMS training programs provide OMS-based exposure to head and neck surgery. This exposure not only improves our surgical prowess, but, owing to the significant comorbidities that routinely accompany these patients, we further our ability to understand and apply medicine, refine our airway expertise, and interact with other providers.

This issue of *Oral and Maxillofacial Surgery Clinics of North America* presents contributions from a number of experts within our specialty whom I deeply respect. It not only honors many of the pioneers of OMS-based neck surgery but is also an expression of a vital up-and-coming generation of OMS head and neck surgeons. The issue begins with a discussion of contemporary imaging modalities used in evaluating neck masses. Subsequent articles address pediatric patients, soft tissue tumors as well as neck masses from a variety of etiologies including infectious, hematopoietic, endocrine, salivary, vascular, and metastatic disease.

Atlas Oral Maxillofacial Surg Clin N Am 23 (2015) ix–x
1061-3315/15/$ - see front matter © 2015 Published by Elsevier Inc.
http://dx.doi.org/10.1016/j.cxom.2014.12.001

The issue concludes with a discussion of the reconstruction of cervical defects.

Thanks

I want to express thanks to all who have assisted in this work, from past and current colleagues to residents who continue to challenge me. I am also greatly indebted to my wife and parents. Last, thanks be to God for allowing me the privilege of treating His children and allowing me to enjoy it so much!

David E. Webb, Maj, USAF, DC
Department of Oral and Maxillofacial Surgery
David Grant USAF Medical Center
Travis AFB, CA, USA

David Grant USAF Medical Center
101 Bodin Circle/SGDD
Travis AFB, CA 94535, USA

E-mail address:
david.webb.5@us.af.mil

Contemporary Use of Imaging Modalities in Neck Mass Evaluation

John N. St.J Blythe, FRCS (OMFS), FDS, RCS (Eng), FRCS (Eng) [a,*],
Oliver J. Pearce, FRCR, MBBS [b], Elizabeth A. Tilley, FRCR, FRCP [b],
Peter A. Brennan, MD, FRCS, FRCSI, FDS [a]

KEYWORDS

- Neck mass • Neck ultrasonography • Neck computer tomogram • Neck magnetic resonance imaging • Diagnosis

KEY POINTS

- The incidence of new cases of head and neck cancer in the United Kingdom is approximately 8100.
- In most patients presenting with neck masses, the diagnosis is benign.
- The clinical effectiveness and efficiency of separating malignant from benign not only has a significant impact for the patient but also economic benefit to health care providers.

Introduction

A patient presenting to clinic with a neck lump is a common scenario for oral and maxillofacial/head and neck surgeons. In this article, the diagnosis and management of common and important neck masses are discussed, with particular focus on the various roles of imaging. The focus is on adult neck lumps. Thyroid lumps and pediatric cervical swellings are excluded from this discussion. More emphasis is placed on the practicalities of imaging and management rather than the provision of an exhaustive list of differential diagnoses.

In our department, 900 new patients present to a designated 1-stop neck lump clinic annually. The service allows regional general medical and dental practitioners the opportunity for rapid referral of patients with neck lumps of concerning origin. Most patients attending the 1-stop clinic receive senior clinician assessment, coupled with immediate ultrasonography (US) and cytologic investigations, where indicated. By the end of the patient's visit to the clinic, the patient receives a preliminary diagnosis and a scheduled investigative time scale. After a contemporary departmental audit, approximately 12% of these new referrals are diagnosed as malignant.

Approximately 8100 new cases of head and neck cancer are registered in England annually.[1] Seventy-three percent of patients in the United Kingdom with head and neck cancer are referred from primary care under the urgent or 2-week referral system.[2] In the United Kingdom, the incidence of cancer with unknown primary is 10,000, many of these present as cervical malignancy with undiagnosed primary origin.[3]

In our clinic, most presenting neck lumps are benign, with reactive or suppurative lymphadenopathy, lipomata, and superficial and deep cervical cysts. Benign disease of the parotid tail and submandibular and sublingual glands are also common presentations. Less frequent referrals relate to variations of normal anatomy: a prominent carotid bulb or a spinous process of cervical vertebra or a cervical rib.

The radiology team has an important role in the assessment and diagnosis of neck lumps. In particular, the ability of the radiologist to identify cancer spread and accurately stage malignancy is a key and often pivotal role in influencing treatment at the multidisciplinary team meeting. This situation has reflected the advances across the field of imaging in recent times. In this article, the imaging modalities available are reviewed, highlighting their merits and hurdles of use, and, second, the common and significant neck lumps presenting to our head and neck clinic are reviewed.

Anatomic classification of the neck

Cervical Lymphatic Classification

The extensive lymphatic system in the head and neck provides a physiologic mechanism for channeling fluid, cells, and protein from the interstitium into the systemic circulation. There are approximately 300 lymph nodes within this region, which account for 40% of the total body lymph nodes. An understanding of the head and neck lymphatic system is needed in the management of patients with head and neck cancer with regional metastasis. Lymphatics in the neck have been classified into superficial and deep systems (Fig. 1). The superficial system arising in the reticular dermis and superficial cervical fascia and the deep lymphatic circulation functions beneath the investing layer of the deep cervical fascia (Table 1). The American Head and Neck Society and American

Funding Support: Not applicable.

The authors have nothing to disclose.

[a] Department of Oral and Maxillofacial Surgery, Queen Alexandra Hospital, Cosham, Portsmouth PO6 3LY, UK

[b] Department of Radiology, Queen Alexandra Hospital, Cosham, Portsmouth PO6 3LY, UK

* Corresponding author.

E-mail address: Jnstj.blythe@btopenworld.com

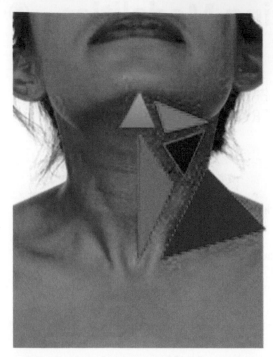

Fig. 1 Anterior and posterior triangles of the neck. Anterior: submental (*blue*), submandibular (*green*), muscular (*orange*), carotid (*purple*); posterior (*red*).

Academy of Otolaryngology—Head and Neck Surgery organized the cervical lymphatic system into separate levels, reflecting patterns of drainage (Fig. 2, Table 2). This division provides reproducible anatomic localization for both surgeon and radiologist.

Consultation appointment

With the space constraints of this article, the full history taking and examination process are not considered. However, the importance of targeted questions relevant to diagnosis must be highlighted. The fundamental aim of the clinic is to identify the malignant conditions from most referrals that prove benign. Patients presenting with an undiagnosed malignancy may have been suffering local, regional, and systematic symptoms associated with local tumor behavior and metastatic and paraneoplastic effects. In addition, questions about B symptoms in suspected lymphoma are recommended. A careful social history analyzing tobacco and alcohol habits and details of past sexual practice assigns a level of risk to the patient.

Specific questions on renal function and allergy are required before referring for radiologic investigations requiring intravenous contrast. Inherited and acquired coagulopathies need to be identified before invasive sampling. We have found that increasingly more patients attending clinic report taking new-generation antiplatelets (eg, prasugrel, ticagrelor, clopidogrel). These antiplatelets can be easily overlooked but require appropriate discussion with hematology colleagues before investigative procedures and treatment.

A routine head and neck examination should be performed, which should include an oral examination and flexible nasal endoscopy. Clues from the history may encourage the clinician to examine the chest, axillae, abdomen, and nervous system.

Findings and recommendations from the Eighth Annual Review of Data Analysis of Head and Neck Oncology[2] showed that only 80% of patients had TNM cancer staging and 66% performance status recorded at the time of multidisciplinary team discussion. The initial consultation is an ideal time to start collecting this information.

Imaging modalities in the assessment of neck lumps

Radiology is continually and rapidly advancing and forms a critical component of the diagnostic pathway for investigating neck lumps. Faster image acquisition, improved resolution, and expanding software capabilities all contribute to more detailed and more informative imaging.

The main imaging modalities used in the assessment of lumps presenting in the head and neck are US, computed tomography (CT), magnetic resonance imaging (MRI), and positron emission tomography (PET). An overview of their strengths and weaknesses is provided in Table 3, with guidance related to image acquisition.

Ultrasonography

US is commonly the first-line imaging modality for assessing neck lumps. It is a quick, well-tolerated examination, which is widely available and offers a high spatial resolution without the use of ionizing radiation. Furthermore, US allows real-time guidance for fine-needle aspiration (FNA) cytology (FNAC) and core biopsy when a tissue sample is required. The main disadvantages of US are that it is limited to relatively superficial structures and is user dependent, with a high level of expertise required for the assessment of neck disease. Image quality is improved if good neck extension can be achieved (Fig. 3).

US evaluation of a neck lump is often sufficient to reassure the patient and referring clinician of a benign cause. Common benign skin and subcutaneous lesions encountered in the neck include reactive lymph nodes, sebaceous cysts, and lipomas (Fig. 4), many of which can be confidently diagnosed on US, negating the need for more expensive cross-sectional imaging or unnecessary surgery.

A focused US examination can also be a useful problem-solving tool. In the setting of head and neck cancer, cross-sectional imaging may show a borderline enlarged lymph node. Deciding whether it is pathologic or reactive can have implications for treatment options. Because of its high spatial resolution, US is able to assess the internal architecture of a lymph node in conjunction with its size measurements. Real-time use of power Doppler sonography provides additional information, with normal or reactive nodes tending to show hilar flow (Fig. 5) whereas metastatic nodes show peripheral or mixed vascularity.[4]

A meta-analysis published in 2007[5] comparing US, US-guided FNAC (USgFNAC), CT, and MRI for the detection of cervical lymph node metastases found that USgFNAC had the greatest accuracy, followed by US, with CT and MRI performing less well.

A relatively recent adjunct to a standard US examination is the use of sonoelastography. Sonoelastography measures the elasticity of a tissue, using either internal or external forces, and works on the principle that malignant lesions are stiffer than benign tissue.[6] Although some promising results have been seen in the evaluation of thyroid lumps, the role of sonoelastography in the investigation of salivary gland tumors and cervical lymphadenopathy is less convincing.

Table 1   Cervical triangles: boundaries and contents

Cervical Triangle	Boundaries	Contents
Anterior		
Submental	Neck midline Lower border of mandible Anterior belly of digastric muscle	Submental vessels uniting with anterior jugular vein Level Ia lymph nodes
Submandibular	Lower border of mandible Anterior belly and digastric Posterior belly of digastric muscle	Facial vessels Level Ib lymph nodes Submandibular gland Marginal mandibular branch of facial nerve Hypoglossal nerve

Carotid	Mid third of sternomastoid muscle
	   (anterior margin)
	Posterior belly of digastric muscle
	Superior belly of omohyoid
		Bifurcation of common carotid artery
		Carotid branches (superior thyroid, lingual, facial, occipital,
		   ascending pharyngeal)
		Internal jugular vein and tributaries (superior thyroid, lingual,
		   common facial, ascending pharyngeal, occipital)
		Sympathetic trunk
		Vagus nerve
		Hypoglossal nerve
		Cervical plexus
		Spinal accessory nerve
		Level II/III lymph nodes
		Upper larynx/lower pharynx

Muscular	Lower third of sternocleidomastoid
	   (anterior margin)
	Superior belly of omohyoid
	Median line of neck (hyoid to sternum)
		Carotid sheath (common carotid artery, internal jugular vein,
		   vagus nerve, sympathetic trunk)
		Ansa cervicalis
		Inferior thyroid artery and vein
		Esophagus
		Thyroid gland
		Trachea
		Lower part of larynx
		Recurrent laryngeal nerve
		Level II/III lymph nodes

Posterior	Anterior border of trapezius Middle third of clavicle posterior border of SCM	Transverse cervical vessels Distal part of subclavian artery Suprascapular artery Lower part of external jugular vein Level V lymph nodes Spinal accessory nerve Cervical plexus Phrenic nerve (C3,4,5)

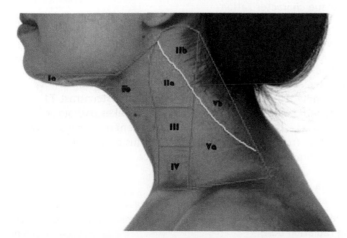

Fig. 2   The American Head and Neck Society and American Academy of Otolaryngology—Head and Neck Surgery classification of cervical lymph nodes shown on a profile view of the neck.

In 2004, the National Institute for Clinical Excellence published *Improving Outcomes in Head and Neck Cancer—The Manual*,[7] which made the recommendation that "diagnostic clinics should be established for patients with neck lumps." These clinics take many forms but usually consist of a US list and rapid cytologic analysis running in parallel with the surgical clinic.

Computed Tomography

If US evaluation is inconclusive or raises concerns regarding more extensive disease, then cross-sectional imaging is required. CT is readily available and relatively cheap, although it entails an ionizing radiation burden. Although it provides excellent anatomic and bony detail, CT is limited in its soft tissue resolution, most noticeably in patients with little body fat to separate muscles from nodes and vascular structures. CT is also susceptible to metallic streak artifact from dental restorations (Fig. 6), and, although acquisition on modern

Table 2 The American Head and Neck Society and American Academy of Otolaryngology–Head and Neck Surgery classification of cervical lymph nodes

Level	Anatomic Site	Draining Source
IA	Submental triangle	Lips, chin, nasal tip, incisors/canines
IB	Submandibular triangle	Cheek, premolar and molar teeth, anterior tongue
IIA	Base of skull to upper border of hyoid bone: anterior to SAN	Oropharynx, anterior and posterior tongue
IIB	Base of skull to upper border of hyoid bone: posterior to SAN	Oropharynx, parotid
III	Upper border of hyoid bone to upper border of cricoid	Oropharynx, larynx
IV	Upper border of cricoid to upper border of clavicle	Oropharynx, larynx, upper thorax
VA	Posterior triangle: anterior to SAN	Occiput and scalp
VB	Posterior triangle: distal to SAN	Occiput and scalp
VI	Lower border of hyoid to suprasternal notch. Lateral border is common carotid artery	Thyroid gland, larynx, piriform sinus, esophagus

Abbreviation: SAN, spinal accessory nerve.
Adapted from Robbins KT, Shaha AR, Medina JE, et al. Consensus statement on the classification and terminology of neck dissection. Arch Otolaryngol Head Neck Surg 2008;134(5):536–8.

scanners is rapid, images are still prone to movement artifact, such as swallowing.

Intravenous iodinated contrast administration is required for optimal CT evaluation of the neck, assuming good renal function. This practice causes an adverse reaction in 5% to 8% of patients, with life-threatening allergic reactions in 0.1%.[8] Intravenous iodinated contrast is also contraindicated in certain patients with renal failure. The rate of administration

Table 3 Imaging modalities: summary of strengths, weaknesses, and practical tips

Modality	Strengths	Weaknesses	Tips and Technique

US	Cheap and available
	Patient friendly:
	    No safety issues
	    Patient does not have to lie completely still
	    No ionizing radiation
	High-resolution real-time imaging
	US-guided fine-needle aspiration and biopsy
		Operator dependent; neck US best performed by specialist head and neck radiologist
		Limited depth penetration
		Limited visualization of bony structures
			Patient scanned with neck extended
			High-frequency probe (8–12 MHz)

CT	Available
	Patient friendly:
	    Quick (<5 min to complete scan)
	    Not claustrophobic
	    No breath hold required
	    Kyphotic patients can be scanned
	Single supine scan with volumetric data allowing multiplanar reconstruction
	Good anatomic localization
	Excellent bony detail
	Can simultaneously image the chest for staging in the setting of malignancy
		Uses ionizing radiation
		Requires intravenous iodinated contrast for optimum visualization of structures in the neck
		Image quality degraded by artifact from dental amalgam and swallowing
		Limited soft tissue characterization
			Scan during quiet breathing
			Slow intravenous injection of contrast (100 mL injected at 1 mL/s and scanned at 100 s) for arterial, venous. and soft tissue enhancement

MRI	Excellent soft tissue characterization
	No ionizing radiation
		Expensive and less readily available
		Less patient friendly than CT:
		    Safety issues with implants (eg, pacemaker)
		    Longer scan time (typically 30 min)
		    Scan quality degraded by motion artifact
		    Claustrophobia can be an issue
		    Unable to scan kyphotic patients
			Scan with quiet breathing
			Fat-saturated postcontrast T1 sequence makes pathologic enhancement more conspicuous
			Acquire diffusion-weighted sequence

PET/CT	Provides functional data regarding metabolic activity of the primary tumor and any metastatic disease Wider scan range (typically skull base to mid thighs or whole body)	Expensive and limited availability High ionizing radiation dose	

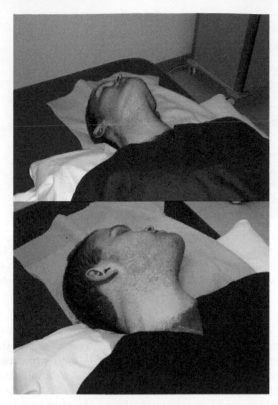

Fig. 3 US position. The correct patient positioning for a neck US scan is shown in these photographs. (*Top*) The pillow is positioned under the shoulders, allowing the neck to be extended. If the patient is unable to extend their neck sufficiently, then, limited views are obtained. (*Bottom*) The patient first turns their chin away from the scanner, allowing greater access to the right neck. Turning the patient's chin toward the scanner allows optimal examination of the left neck.

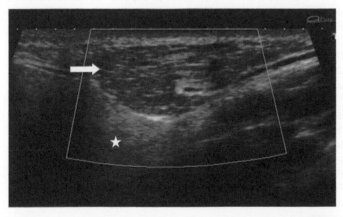

Fig. 4 Lipoma over parotid. A 42-year-old male patient presented with a soft palpable lump in the region of the right parotid gland. US with Doppler (note the *green box*) showed the typical US features of a lipoma (*solid arrow*) overlying the right parotid gland (*star*). The lipoma had an elliptical shape, appeared mildly hypoechoic compared with the surrounding fat, and contained multiple fine echogenic lines running parallel to the skin surface. No appreciable internal vascularity was identified. The patient was reassured and discharged from clinic.

of contrast and time between administering the contrast and acquiring the scan can be altered to enable optimal visualization of different structures. For general neck lump assessment, a slow injection rate (1 mL/s) with a delayed scan at 100 seconds is recommended. At this point, there is adequate contrast within both the arterial and venous system to allow accurate interpretation. In the setting of head and neck cancer, this slow injection rate and delayed phase of scanning also result in improved delineation of tumor edge compared with a faster injection rate and earlier scan time (Fig. 7).[9] More rapid injection rates with earlier scan times may be appropriate if the neck lump is believed to be related to the arterial system, for example an aneurysm.

CT perfusion (CTP) is a comparatively new technique used in the evaluation of malignant neck lumps. It is a method for assessing neoangiogenesis and is used in some centers to detect, stage, and predict the behaviors of head and neck tumors, as well as to assess postchemoradiotherapy response.[10] CTP requires a fast injection rate and the acquisition of repeated scans every few seconds. CTP allows parameters such as blood flow, blood volume, and permeability surface to be calculated, all of which are typically high in squamous cell carcinomas. The role of CTP in other tumors, particularly parotid neoplasms, is still under investigation. CTP is not widely available in the United Kingdom, and repeated acquisitions result in an increased ionizing radiation dose.

MRI

MRI has the major advantage of improved soft tissue resolution compared with CT (Fig. 8). However, it requires a longer acquisition time, typically 30 minutes, and requires the patient to be motionless during scan acquisition. MRI is also contra-indicated in certain patients, most commonly because of insertion of non–MRI-compatible pacemakers, and is not easily tolerated by claustrophobic patients. In the setting of sepsis and airway compromise, the patient may be deemed too unstable to undertake a long investigation with limited access to the patient for monitoring.

For the complete assessment of neck lumps, precontrast and postcontrast sequences are required to analyze the enhancement pattern of the mass. Because both gadolinium-based contrast agents and fat are high signal (white) on T1-weighted imaging, fat-suppressed T1-weighted postcontrast sequences ensure that pathologic enhancement is more conspicuous.

The quality of diffusion-weighted imaging (DWI), which is based on the free diffusion of water molecules, has improved such that it is useful in the analysis of neck lumps. Hyper-cellular tumors, such as lymphoma and squamous cell carcinoma, and pus within an abscess tend to show restricted diffusion. Benign lesions and inflammatory change typically show free diffusion of water.[11] DWI is often particularly useful in the clinical setting of head and neck cancer recurrence, in which clinical examination and conventional imaging may not be able to distinguish tumor recurrence from posttreatment change. Salivary gland neoplasms are more heterogeneous, with overlap in diffusion characteristics between benign and malignant lesions.

Similar to CTP, dynamic contrast-enhanced MRI is being used in some centers to predict the response of head and neck cancers to radiotherapy. Preliminary results have shown that in

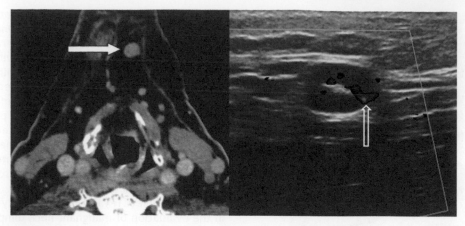

Fig. 5 Borderline submental node. A 76-year-old male patient had a previous history of tongue base carcinoma treated with chemo-radiotherapy. He presented after a 6-year disease-free period with mandibular pain. On examination, he had a palpable submental lymph node. No mandibular abnormality was seen on CT, but there was an indeterminate, prominent submental node, measuring 8 mm (*solid arrow*). US confirmed a normal lymph node structure with an echogenic hilum and hilar blood flow (*outlined arrow*), enabling a confident diagnosis of a reactive node.

T3/T4 tumors, those with higher blood flows and blood volumes respond better to treatment, although more patients are required for validation.[12]

Positron Emission Tomography

PET is a functional imaging tool, which has a limited but important role in the evaluation of neck lumps. The most widely used radiotracer is [[18]]fluorodeoxyglucose (FDG), which is a radiolabeled glucose analogue taken up by metabolically active cells. Because of the increased levels of aerobic glycolysis and the increased expression of glucose-transporter

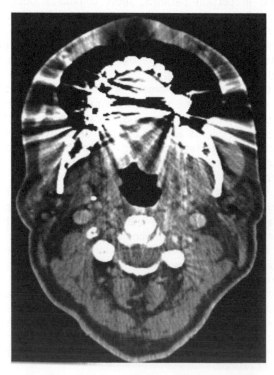

Fig. 6 Metallic streak artifact. Metallic streak artifact throughout the oral cavity secondary to dental restorations is common and obscures views of the oral cavity.

proteins in malignant cells, FDG accumulates in malignant lesions, showing up as hot spots (Fig. 9).[13] A quantitative and reproducible scale of relative FDG uptake can be applied to the hot spot using the standardized uptake value (SUV). The SUV takes into account the amount of FDG injected and the patient's size, such that if all injected FDG is retained and uniformly distributed, the SUV is 1 g/mL, irrespective of the patient size and amount of FDG injected.[14]

PET imaging is usually combined with a low-dose CT scan, which is used for anatomic colocalization. It is essential to correlate that areas of uptake correspond with disease as physiologic hot spots are encountered, most commonly in brown fat and recently active muscles. More recently, the advantages of PET/MR have been investigated.

In clinical practice, the main applications of PET/CT are to stage head and neck cancer when there is concern regarding distant disease and to search for an unknown primary lesion. PET/CT and MRI are also considered superior to standard CT at detecting tumor recurrence and second primary lesions with PET/CT, offering the added advantage of a systemic evaluation. The current recommendation from the British Association of Head and Neck Oncologists is that MRI and PET/CT should be used when recurrence of head and neck cancer is suspected.[15]

Although PET provides important functional information, it is a low-resolution technique and is not always reliable at detecting metastatic lesions smaller than 1 cm. False-negative scans can also be encountered in the setting of necrosis, as is seen with some squamous cell carcinoma nodal metastases (Fig. 10). In addition to false-negative scans, false-positive PET/CT results are encountered as a result of an overlap in the uptake characteristics between inflammatory and neoplastic lesions.

Specific neck lumps

In this section, the imaging and management of both common and significant neck swellings presenting to our department are discussed. This is not an exhaustive series of clinical scenarios but is aimed to show the imaging algorithms and diagnostic features on imaging and to address relevant controversies.

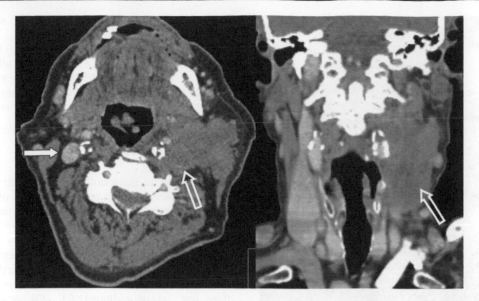

Fig. 7 Internal jugular vein invasion nodal disease. A 68-year-old female patient presented with a large left nodal mass extending throughout the left neck. The slow-injection delayed-phase imaging optimized delineation of the tumor edge and ensured contrast in both the arterial and venous system. This technique allowed visualization of the normal right internal jugular vein (*solid arrow*). The left internal jugular vein did not opacify because of involvement of the vascular sheath by the tumor (*outlined arrows*). This finding has important surgical implications. The loss of the fat plane between the tumor and the left sternocleidomastoid muscle indicated infiltration.

Infections Involving the Neck

Rapidly spreading infection into the neck is a common sequel to severe dental infection and peritonsillar abscesses. Acute bacterial submandibular sialadenitis may also present with upper cervical swelling. Successful management is initially based on a sound history and clinical examination. The cause and tissue space involvement can often be identified on clinical grounds. However, there are occasions when the clinical features fail to allow a distinction between surgically drainable abscess and cellulitis. Imaging modalities assist in confirming the cause of sepsis (eg, panoral radiograph) and tissue space involvement (US/CT).

When acute infection presents as a neck lump, there is soft tissue edema and thickening, which limits the penetration of US, often resulting in inadequate views. This factor can introduce an unnecessary delay in the diagnostic pathway, because CT is required. Unless the infection is clinically confined to the skin or subcutaneous soft tissues, CT with

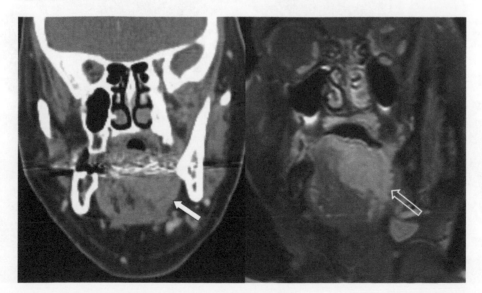

Fig. 8 Improved visualization of tongue lesion with MRI. A 71-year-old female patient presented with lymphadenopathy in the neck and had a large tongue lesion on examination. Initial CT partially visualized the left tongue tumor (*solid arrow*), but the superior soft tissue characterization available with MRI enabled more accurate delineation of the tumor (*outlined arrow*).

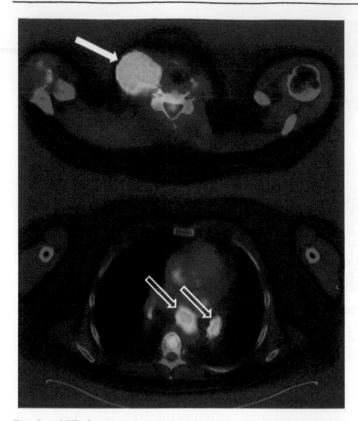

Fig. 9 PET of neck and mediastinal hilar nodes. Malignant lesions show uptake of FDG as hot spots on the PET scan. This patient presented with a right neck mass. He had a right tonsillar primary squamous cell carcinoma, with widespread lymphadenopathy in the neck (*solid arrow*) and chest (*outlined arrows*).

intravenous contrast extending from the skull base to the carina should be the first-line investigation.

The major diagnostic benefit of CT over US is to diagnose the presence and extent of a deep, clinically occult collection (Fig. 11). CT can also aid in assessment of the airway and exclude jugular vein thrombosis. In the absence of a focal fluid collection, conservative management may be the preferred strategy (Fig. 12).

Parotid Tail Swelling

Acute bacterial sialadenitis is a clinical diagnosis requiring medical management, and imaging is often not indicated. When there is clinical suspicion of an obstructive cause or concern of suppuration, then, US is the first-line investigation. This modality has excellent sensitivity and specificity for identification of intraglandular and extraglandular ductal dilatation and sialolith formation. If further insight into the condition is required, the second-line imaging includes plain films (eg, lateral oblique), CT, MRI, or conventional sialography. Choice is often dependent on local availability and expertise. In the rare case of a parotid abscess, US-guided drainage may obviate surgical drainage.

Parotid gland neoplasia is regularly referred into our fast-track neck lump clinic from primary care. After a comprehensive consultation, the imaging algorithm in Fig. 13 is followed.

US is the primary investigation of choice for a discrete parotid lump and can be used to ascertain whether the mass is solitary or multiple. Certain parotid diseases may have characteristic US features. For example, a pleomorphic adenoma may be well defined, with a lobulated outline and posterior acoustic enhancement, whereas a Warthin tumor typically has a partially cystic appearance and may be multiple. However, there is considerable overlap in the appearances of benign and malignant diseases, for example between a low-grade well-differentiated mucoepidermoid carcinoma and a pleomorphic adenoma.[4] Thus, the main value in performing US is to guide

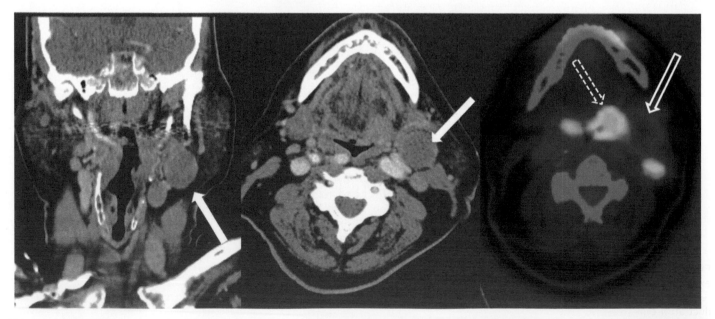

Fig. 10 Determining a necrotic node: CT versus PET. Coronal (*left*) and axial (*middle*) slices from diagnostic CT show a large left level II necrotic lymph node (*solid arrows*) and less apparent asymmetrical enhancement involving the left tongue base. PET/CT confirmed the presence of a tongue base primary tumor (*dashed arrow*) but showed poor uptake in the large necrotic node (*outlined arrow*).

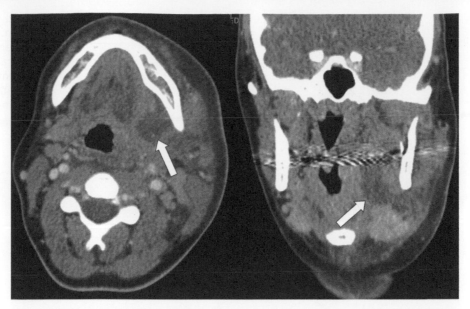

Fig. 11 A previously fit and well 35-year-old white woman presented with a 2-day history of left facial pain and rapidly progressing floor of mouth and upper neck swelling after a left mandibular first molar extraction. On examination, the patient was pyrexial, tachypneic, and tachycardic. The patient had partial trismus and tense swelling of the left floor of mouth. In addition, the patient had erythema and fluctuant swelling associated with the left submandibular triangle. CT confirmed a focal fluid density adjacent to the lingual cortex of the left mandible and in continuity with the tooth extraction socket. A sublingual and submandibular abscess was diagnosed, and the patient received intravenous fluid resuscitation and intravenous empirical antibiotics compliant with local antimicrobial prescribing guidelines. Under general anesthesia, the submandibular and sublingual abscess was drained via the Hilton technique, and corrugated rubber drains placed. The lower extraction socket was explored, followed by debridement and irrigation. A microbial sample was sent for further culture and sensitivity. The patient recovered well and was discharged 2 days later.

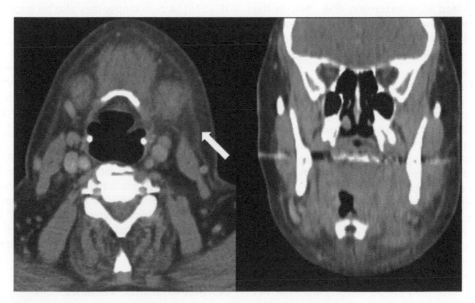

Fig. 12 A 43-year-old Asian man with type 2 diabetes mellitus presented with a 3-day history of left upper neck swelling and pain. On examination, the patient was apyrexial and hemodynamically stable. The patient had a hot and tender swelling in the left submandibular region. On intraoral inspection, there was tenderness of the submandibular gland, and no saliva could be expressed from the left Wharton duct after bimanual massage. CT showed inflammatory stranding within the left submandibular gland and subcutaneous soft tissues with thickening of the platysma. No focal fluid collection to indicate an abscess was identified. No calcification or dilatation was identified in the Wharton duct. A diagnosis of acute submandibular sialadenitis was made. The patient received intravenous coamoxiclav and was discharged 3 days later, once the swelling had resolved.

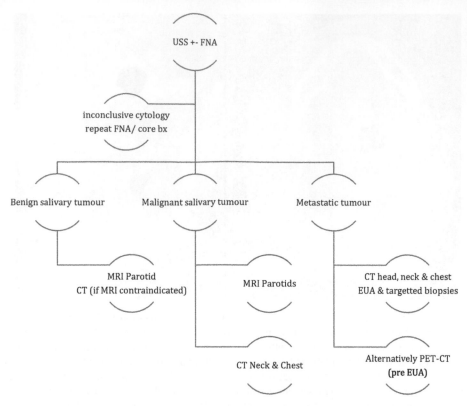

Fig. 13 Parotid tumor algorithm.

FNA for a cytologic diagnosis. However, a dilemma exists if the FNAC result is reported as inconclusive. We have found excellent diagnostic yields after a repeat FNAC in more than 90% of cases.[16]

If a parotid mass cannot be visualized in its entirety on US, an MRI scan is useful to show its location and, in particular, whether there is any deep lobe extension (Fig. 14). In the setting of suspected recurrence of pleomorphic adenoma, a heavily T2-weighted MRI sequence aids in localization of all recurrent nodules.

Benign Neck Swellings

Some of the most common benign neck swellings are listed in the following sections. As discussed earlier, common superficial benign neck lumps can also be confidently diagnosed at US, obviating cross-sectional imaging or an unnecessary biopsy. Lipomas and sebaceous cysts are the most frequently encountered lesions in our clinical practice.

Simple cystic lesions visualized with US can usually be considered benign, but particular care must be taken when a cystic mass is found in level II. In a young patient, this mass is most likely to be a second branchial cleft cyst, but in an older patient, a necrotic malignant node can look identical. FNA or biopsy must be performed. We have encountered a lesion consistent with a branchial cleft cyst on imaging and FNA, but with a histologic diagnosis of squamous cell carcinoma after surgical excision (Fig. 15).

Malignant Masses

Clinically hard, irregular and fixed neck masses that are increasing in size are concerning for malignancy. Most patients with these masses present to our neck lump clinic, where a full history and clinical examination are performed before neck US, with US-guided FNA as appropriate. If the primary site of malignancy is obvious after clinical examination and flexible nasoendoscopy, then, urgent head, neck, and chest CT is performed for local and distant staging (Fig. 16). A core biopsy may also be necessary if a larger tissue sample is required, commonly in the setting of suspected lymphoma.

If the primary lesion is shown poorly with CT, contrast-enhanced MRI is performed (Fig. 17). Areas of concern on the scan provide targets for subsequent examination and biopsies under anesthesia. After imaging and cytology or histology, the case is presented at the weekly head and neck multidisciplinary team meeting and available treatment options discussed.

Locally, if lymphoma is suspected, either from the history, clinical examination, or US findings, then, staging CT to cover the neck, chest, abdomen, and pelvis is performed, although, in some centers, PET/CT may be the preferred initial investigation for suspected lymphoma. PET/CT is also the preferred initial cross-sectional imaging modality for an unknown primary tumor presenting with confirmed metastatic nodal disease in the neck.

Normal Anatomic Variants

Several normal anatomic variants may present as a neck lump, and US assists diagnosis of most of these. In our practice, commonly seen neck lumps referred to the urgent 1-stop neck lump clinic include ectatic carotid bulbs, normal submandibular glands (Fig. 18), prominent cervical spine transverse processes, and cervical ribs (Fig. 19).

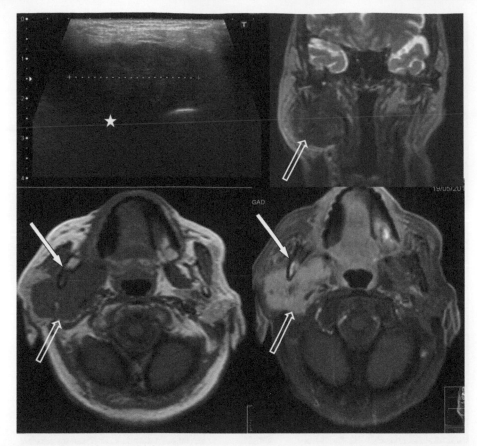

Fig. 14 Parotid mass US and MRI. A 63-year-old female patient presented with a 6-week history of a painless parotid swelling, globus pharyngeus, and paresthesia of the right side of the lower lip and chin. Extraoral examination showed a 4-cm × 3-cm firm mass and paresthesia in the distribution of the right inferior alveolar nerve. On intraoral examination, asymmetry of the palatine tonsils caused by medial displacement of the right tonsil was shown. (*Top left*) US shows a heterogeneous mass (dimensions) involving the superficial aspect of the parotid gland, but the deep extent is poorly visualized. FNA confirmed adenocarcinoma. (*Top right*) Coronal T2 sequence shows that the heterogeneous intermediate-signal and low-signal mass extends to the deep lobe of the right parotid gland. (*Bottom images*) T1 precontrast and T1 postcontrast fat-saturated images confirm a large enhancing mass involving the superficial and deep aspects of the right parotid gland, with extension into the inferior alveolar nerve canal and adjacent abnormal marrow signal in the ramus of the mandible. The patient underwent a right total parotidectomy with a lip split mandibulotomy, selective neck dissection, and postoperative radiotherapy. Histology showed a low-grade adenocarcinoma.

Practical challenges

Psychological Barriers (Claustrophobia)

Claustrophobia and imaging-related anxiety are commonly encountered problems in patients at the time of scanning and can be addressed on several levels. At the consultation appointment, the psychosocial history may highlight at-risk patients and allow 1 or a combination of the following measures to ensure a compliant patient to both first attend the imaging appointment and second remain motionless during the scan to optimize image quality. The provision of patient education leaflets and relevant Web site addresses allows the patient to learn about the imaging process in the comfort of their own home. For some patients, a preliminary visit to the CT or MRI scanner helps reassure them and reduces anxiety. From a pharmacology level, mild oral sedation with benzodiapezines (eg, diazepam 2 mg the night before and on the morning of the scan) is sufficient to settle anxiety, without the danger of oversedation and respiratory depression. Aromatherapy and acupuncture can also be considered helpful options. Imaging companies have also adapted scanner design to improve patient experience. Simple measures such as patient entry into the scanner feet first, runway lights, cooling fans, and audio speakers have reduced anxieties.

Physical Barriers (Obesity)

Narrow-bore MRI and CT scanners have made scanning problematic for obese patients. Historically, scanners had a bore of 60 cm, but manufacturers have addressed this challenge by increasing the bore to 70 cm and offering open scanners. In addition, the construction of scanners with a lower table set has raised the habitus threshold for scanning.

Nonpalpable Lump

In the time between initial consultation and diagnostics to surgery for open biopsy, the neck lump may have reduced in size and become difficult to palpate. Good communication between surgeon and radiologist ensures that the patient receives further US immediately before the operation, with skin marking to precisely locate the mass.

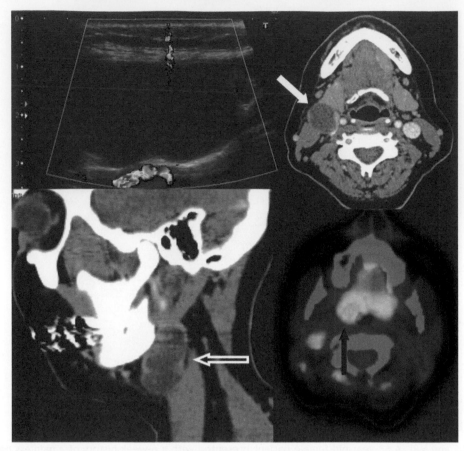

Fig. 15 A 54-year-old male patient presented with a right level II neck mass, which was clinically soft. Head and neck examination was otherwise normal. (*Top left*) US confirmed a largely cystic lesion between the parotid tail and submandibular gland. There was only a small echogenic component and thin septation. FNA did not show malignant cells. (*Top right* and *bottom left*) These appearances were confirmed on CT, and a working diagnosis of branchial cleft cyst made. After surgical excision, histologic diagnosis confirmed squamous cell carcinoma. (*Bottom right*) Subsequent PET/CT diagnosed an occult right tonsillar primary lesion. After multidisciplinary team discussion, the patient received a dental assessment followed by radical radiotherapy to both tonsil bed and neck.

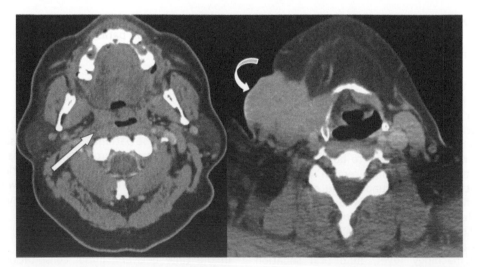

Fig. 16 A 66-year-old white man with a 35-pack-year history presented with a 2-month history of a progressively enlarging asymptomatic neck mass, anorexia, and weight loss. Examination showed a large, hard, and fungating right neck lump and intraorally asymmetrical tonsils. Initial US and core biopsy confirmed metastatic squamous cell carcinoma. Staging neck and chest CT showed an asymmetrically bulky right palatine tonsil consistent with a primary tumor and the metastatic node in right level II. The patient underwent chemo-radiotherapy with cisplatin and 5 fluorouracil (radiotherapy 66 Gy over 33 fractions).

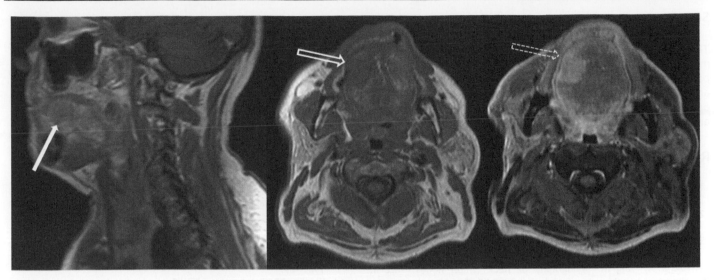

Fig. 17 Although this primary tongue lesion was visible with CT, its margins could not be defined because of a combination of dental streak artifact and poor inherent soft tissue resolution. Precontrast T1 (*left*) and postcontrast T1 fat-saturated (*right*) sequences clearly show a large tongue tumor, which crosses the midline.

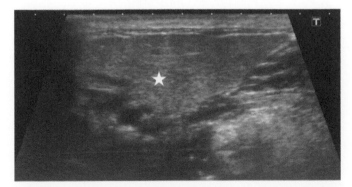

Fig. 18 A 28-year-old female patient was referred via her dentist with a new asymptomatic neck lump. Examination showed mild asymmetry of the submandibular triangles but no obvious mass. The lump indicated by the patient corresponded to a normal submandibular gland after US investigation.

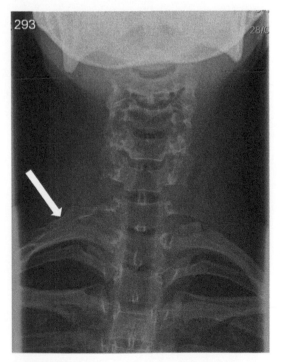

Fig. 19 A 33-year-old female patient presented to the neck lump clinic with a right supraclavicular fossa swelling. Clinically, the swelling was hard and fixed. US did not show a soft tissue abnormality, and the lump corresponded with a cervical rib shown on a plain film.

Summary

The effective and efficient management of a patient with a neck mass in a 1-stop clinic requires a collaborative and harmonious partnership among surgeon, radiologist, and pathologist. In this article, important theoretic and practical issues are discussed to optimize patient care when prescribing, planning, performing, and interpreting imaging for neck disease.

References

1. Cancer statistics registrations, England. Available at: http://www. ons.gov.uk/ons/search/index.html?newquery=mb1.
2. 8th National head and neck cancer audit 2012. Available at: http://www.hscic.gov.uk/clinicalaudits.
3. NICE clinical guideline. 2014. Available at: http://www.nice.org. uk/nicemedia/live/13044/49848/49848.pdf.
4. Ahuja A, Ying M. Sonography of neck lymph nodes. Part II: abnormal lymph nodes. Clin Radiol 2003;58:359—66.
5. De Bondt RB, Nelemans PJ, Hofman PA, et al. Detection of lymph node metastases in head and neck cancer: a meta-analysis comparing US, USgFNAC, CT and MR imaging. Eur J Radiol 2007;64(2):266—72.
6. Yerli H, Yilmaz T, Oztop I. Clinical importance of diastolic sonoelastographic scoring in the management of thyroid nodules. AJNR Am J Neuroradiol 2013;34(3):E27—30. Published October 27, 2011 as 10.3174/ajnr.A2751.
7. National Institute for Clinical Excellence. Guidance on cancer services. Improving outcomes in head and neck cancers—the manual. 2004.
8. Saljoughian M. Intravenous radiocontrast media: a review of allergic reactions. US Pharm 2012;37(5):HS-14—6.
9. Disini L, Connor S. Improved edge delineation using a low-flow and delayed-phase contrast-enhanced protocol for computed tomography imaging of oral cavity and oropharyngeal malignancies. Clin Radiol 2013;68:167—72.
10. Trojanowska A, Trojanowski P, Drop A, et al. Head and neck cancer: value of perfusion CT in depicting primary tumor spread. Med Sci Monit 2012;18(1):CR112—8.
11. Barbero JP, Jiménez IR, Martin Noguerol T, et al. Utility of MRI diffusion techniques in the evaluation of tumors of the head and neck. Cancers (Basel) 2013;5:875—89. http://dx.doi.org/10.3390/cancers5030875.
12. Agrawal S, Awasthi R. An exploratory study into the role of dynamic contrast-enhanced (DCE) MRI metrics as predictors of response in head and neck cancers. Clin Radiol 2012;67:e1—5.
13. Bhatnagar P, Subesinghe M, Patel C, et al. Functional imaging for radiation treatment planning, response assessment, and adaptive therapy in head and neck cancer. Radiographics 2013;33:1909—29.
14. Kinahan PE, Fletcher JW. PET/CT standardized uptake values (SUVs) in clinical practice and assessing response to therapy. Semin Ultrasound CT MR 2010;31(6):496—505. http://dx.doi.org/10.1053/j.sult.2010.10.001.
15. British Association of Head and Neck Oncologists. Head and neck cancer: multidisciplinary guidelines. 4th edition. 2011.
16. Brennan PA, Davies B, Poller D, et al. Fine needle aspiration cytology (FNAC) of salivary gland tumours: repeat aspiration provides further information in cases with an unclear initial cytological diagnosis. Br J Oral Maxillofac Surg 2010. http://dx.doi.org/10.1016/j.bjoms.2008.12.014.

Pediatric Neck Masses

William J. Curtis, DMD, MD [a],*, Sean P. Edwards, DDS, MD [b]

KEYWORDS

- Pediatric neck mass • Thyroglossal duct cyst • Brachial cleft cyst

KEY POINTS

- Most pediatric neck masses are infectious and resolve without intervention.
- Isolated masses less than 2 cm can be observed for 4 to 6 weeks.
- Pediatric histories should address sick contacts and other vectors.
- Atypical mycobacterium, Epstein-Barr virus, cytomegalovirus, human immunodeficiency virus, and toxoplasmosis should be considered for a suspected infectious process not responding to antibiotic therapy.

Introduction

Neck masses in the pediatric population are a common occurrence. Fortunately, 80% to 90% of pediatric neck masses are benign in nature, with the majority stemming from infectious sources. Infectious processes are usually self-limiting or respond to a short course of oral antibiotics. Other less common sources of pediatric neck masses include congenital malformations, benign neoplasms, and rarely malignancies. Although rare, a malignancy should always be considered in the pediatric patient with a neck mass, and at times biopsy may be indicated.

History and physical examination

A thorough history and physical examination are of utmost importance when dealing with pediatric neck masses. Unfortunately symptoms may be difficult to elicit from children, and much of the history must be obtained through parents or caregivers. This requires the clinician to maintain a high index of suspicion and a low threshold for ordering diagnostic studies. Patient cooperation may also limit physical examination, further lending to the need for additional studies. Vital points in a pediatric neck mass history and physical examination along with possible implications include

- Duration
  - Present since birth typically indicates a benign or congenital process; malignant processes are almost never congenital
  - Vascular malformations generally are present at birth and grow with the child
  - Hemangiomas develop shortly after birth with a rapid growth phase
  - New rapidly growing masses are typically infectious
- Constitutional symptoms
  - Fevers and tenderness are typically infectious signs
  - Recent upper respiratory tract infection suggests reactive lymphadenopathy
  - Symptoms such as fever, malaise, and weight loss may suggest malignancy
- Contact with pets or other vectors
  - Cats or cat feces
  - Wild animals
  - Tick bites
  - Contact with sick children or family members
  - Foreign travel
- Location of mass
  - Midline cystic lesions are typically dermoid or thyroglossal duct cysts (TGDC)
  - Lateral neck masses are most commonly reactive lymphadenitis or brachial cleft cysts
- Consistency and relationship to surrounding structures
  - Shotty lymphadenopathy (multiple small lymph nodes that feel like buckshot) typically indicates reactive lymphadenopathy
  - Hard irregular masses, fixed to deep or surrounding structures may indicate malignancy
- Size
  - Cervical lymph nodes up to 1 cm in size are normal in children younger than 12

A thorough history and physical examination should assist the clinician in placing the mass in one of 3 categories: congenital, infectious, or neoplastic. The most common etiologies of each category are summarized in Table 1.

Initial workup

Although there is no high quality evidence to support the workup of pediatric neck masses, there are a few generally accepted guidelines based on expert opinion and observational studies.

[a] Department of Oral & Maxillofacial Surgery, University of Kentucky College of Dentistry, 800 Rose Street D508, Lexington, KY 40536, USA
[b] Department of Pediatric Oral and Maxillofacial Surgery, University of Michigan, 1500 East Medical Center Drive, Ann Arbor, MI 48109, USA
* Corresponding author.
E-mail address: billcurtis2012@gmail.com

Atlas Oral Maxillofacial Surg Clin N Am 23 (2015) 15-20
1061-3315/15/$ - see front matter © 2015 Elsevier Inc. All rights reserved.
http://dx.doi.org/10.1016/j.cxom.2014.10.002

Table 1 Differential diagnosis of neck masses in children

Location	Developmental	Diagnosis Inflammatory/Reactive	Neoplastic
Anterior sternocleidomastoid	Branchial cleft cyst,[a] vascular malformation	Reactive lymphadenopathy,[a] lymphadenitis (viral, bacterial),[a] sternocleidomastoid tumor of infancy	Lymphoma
Midline	Thyroglossal duct cyst,[a] dermoid cyst[a]	—	Thyroid tumor
Occipital	Vascular malformation	Reactive lymphadenopathy,[a] lymphadenitis[a]	Metastatic lesion
Preauricular	Hemangioma, vascular malformation, type 1 branchial cleft cyst	Reactive lymphadenopathy,[a] lymphadenitis,[a] parotitis,[a] atypical mycobacterium	Pilomatrixoma, salivary gland tumor
Submandibular	Branchial cleft cyst,[a] vascular malformation	Reactive lymphadenopathy,[a] lymphadenitis,[a] atypical mycobacterium	Salivary gland tumor
Submental	Thyroglossal duct cyst,[a] dermoid cyst[a]	Reactive lymphadenopathy,[a] lymphadenitis (viral, bacterial)[a]	—
Supraclavicular	Vascular malformation	—	Lymphoma,[a] metastatic lesion

[a] Type of lesions that are more commonly found in that location.
From Meier JD, Grimmer JF. Evaluation and management of neck masses in children. Am Fam Physician 2014;89(5):354; with permission.

Laboratory Studies
- Routine complete blood cell counts (CBC) are not recommended as part of the initial workup. They may be considered, however, if enlarged lymph nodes fail to resolve after a course of antibiotics
- CBC may help with suspected malignancy
- *Bartonella henselae* titers may be indicated if cat exposure is suspected
- Epstein-Barr virus, cytomegalovirus, HIV, and toxoplasmosis titers may be considered for a suspected infectious process not responding to antibiotic therapy

Imaging Studies
- Ultrasonography is preferred for an afebrile child
- Ultrasonography should be performed for suspected thyroglossal duct cyst to confirm the presence of a normal thyroid gland
- Computed tomography (CT) with contrast for suspected malignancy or deep neck abscess
- MRI is recommended for vascular malformations
- MRI and CT imaging frequently require sedation in the pediatric population

Initial treatment

As mentioned previously, the most common pediatric neck mass etiology is infectious or inflammatory in nature, which ultimately lends itself to a period of watchful waiting. This recommendation is often necessary to avoid inappropriate or overtreatment of the child but frequently results in anxious parents. Official guidelines published by a national organization for the treatment of pediatric neck masses do not exist, but there are generally accepted treatment principles (Fig. 1).

- Observation for bilateral lymphadenitis, lymph nodes <2 cm without tenderness or erythema

- Empiric antibiotics considered for cervical lymphadenitis with systemic symptoms
- Most common infectious organisms are *Staphylococcus aureus* and group A streptococcus
- 10 day course of cephalexin, amoxicillin/clavulanate, or clindamycin

Biopsy should be considered for several situations:

- Hard, firm, or rubbery mass
- Fixed mass
- Supraclavicular mass
- Lymph node larger than 2 cm
- Persistent enlargement longer than 2 weeks
- Failure to respond to antibiotic therapy
- No decrease in size after 4–6 weeks

Surgical treatment

If surgical intervention is deemed necessary for a mass that is not responding to a waiting period or antibiotic therapy, several points should be kept in mind:

- Lymph node biopsies should always be sent fresh for flow cytometry to rule out lymphoma.
- Cultures should include acid-fast bacterium to rule out atypical mycobacterium infections (immunocompetence is a potential cause of chronic cervical lymphadenitis in children younger than 5 years).

Definitive surgical treatment should be considered for congenital neck masses and benign neoplasms to prevent future problems (superinfection or impingement on adjacent structures). A thorough understanding of embryology and anatomy of the developing region is paramount when undertaking the surgical treatment of these entities.

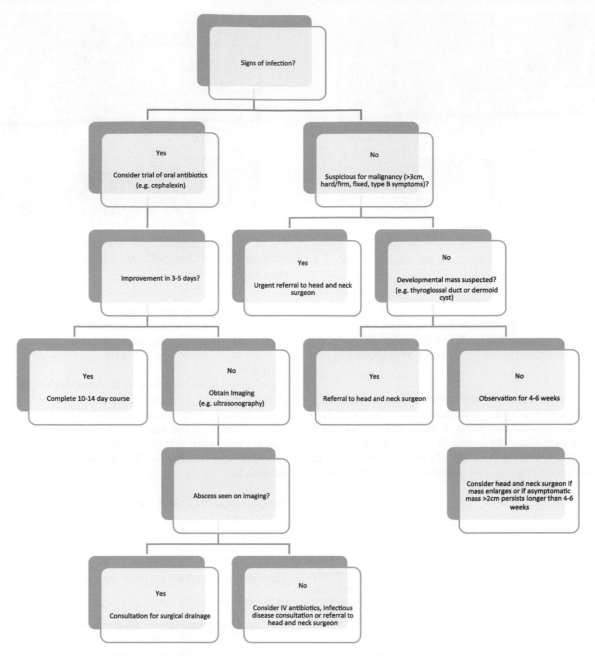

Fig. 1   Workup and management algorithm of pediatric neck masses.

Demonstration of common procedures

Thyroglossal duct cyst excision (Sistrunk procedure)

A normal thyroid should be confirmed with a neck CT or thyroid ultrasound prior to removing a suspected TGDC. If the imaging obtained is abnormal or clinical symptoms of hypothyroidism (constipation, lethargy, developmental and growth delay, excessive somnolence) are present, a radionuclide thyroid scan is indicated to rule out an ectopic thyroid gland.

Step 1
A 2 to 3 cm horizontal skin incision is made in a major skin crease over the cyst. If a draining sinus is present, an ellipse of skin is included in the incision (Fig. 2).

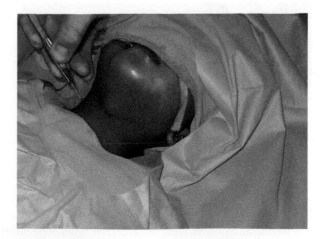

Fig. 2   Mucinous drainage from sinus tract of symptomatic TGDC. (*Courtesy of* Bruce B. Horswell, MD, DDS, MS, Charleston, WV.)

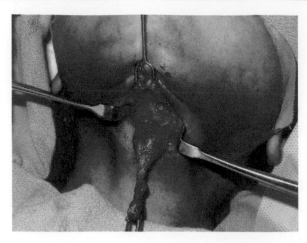

Fig. 3 Thyroglossal duct cyst tethered to the hyoid bone. (*Courtesy of* Bruce B. Horswell, MD, DDS, MS, Charleston, WV.)

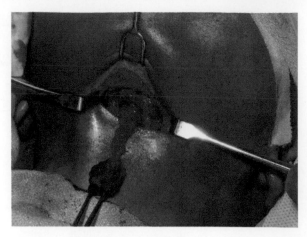

Fig. 5 Tract extending into the base of tongue. Allis clamp grasping the hyoid bone. (*Courtesy of* Bruce B. Horswell, MD, DDS, MS, Charleston, WV.)

Step 2

Blunt dissection proceeds through subcutaneous tissues until the strap muscles are encountered and retracted laterally. At this point, the cyst should be tethered at the hyoid bone (Fig. 3).

Step 3

The hyoid is skeletonized on either side of the cyst using a #15 scalpel, electrocautery and periosteal elevators. Once isolated, bilateral osteotomies using a bone cutter facilitate removal of the cyst from the hyoid. It is vital to remove the central portion of the bone in continuity with the specimen to minimize recurrence (Fig. 4). The remaining segments of hyoid are left free without fixation.

Step 4

A cuff of tongue muscle is removed circumferentially around the tract to the base of the tongue to include the foramen cecum. Some authors advocate placement of a baby Deaver retractor into the vallecula to displace the tongue anteriorly into the surgical field to aid in this maneuver; however, the current authors feel this step is frequently not necessary (Fig. 5). Alternatively, a hand can be placed in the mouth to apply pressure at the foramen cecum to facilitate tracking of

the cyst toward its pharyngeal terminus. The final specimen should include the cyst, the excised central portion of hyoid bone, and tract with tongue musculature (Fig. 6).

Step 5

If the vallecula was entered, it is closed with resorbable suture through the wound created from the approach and leaving the knots buried. The neck wound is closed in layers with approximation of the strap muscles and subcutaneous layer. Skin is closed with 6-0 resorbable suture and covered with skin adhesive and steristrips. Drain placement is typically not necessary.

Second brachial cleft cyst excision

Preoperative assessment generally reveals a ballotable mass in the lateral neck, immediately anterior to the sternocleidomastoid (Fig. 7). A cutaneous fistula may or may not be apparent. A positive history of infection will make excision of

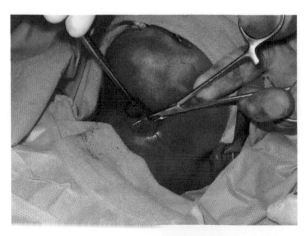

Fig. 4 Hemostat demonstrating skeletonized hyoid bone lateral to the TGDC, which is shown grasped by an Allis clamp. (*Courtesy of* Bruce B. Horswell, MD, DDS, MS, Charleston, WV.)

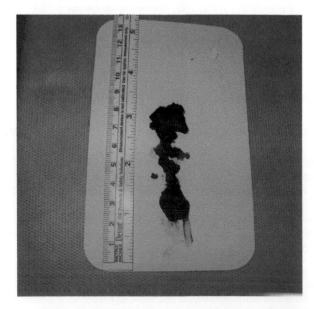

Fig. 6 Entire Thyroglossal duct cyst specimen. (*Courtesy of* Bruce B. Horswell, MD, DDS, MS, Charleston, WV.)

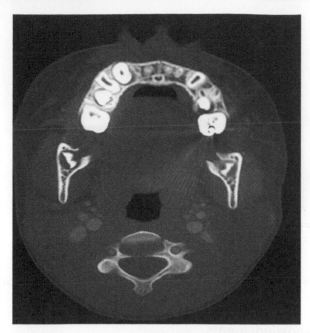

Fig. 7 CT scan showing brachial cleft cyst anterior to the sternocleidomastoid muscle with compression of the internal jugular vein.

the cyst more difficult. Generally, definitive excision is deferred in the setting of acute infection.

Patient preparation

As is the case with most neck surgery, a shoulder roll is placed to aid in extension of the patient's neck. The head is turned to the opposite side and the patient prepared from clavicle to brow (Fig. 8).

Step 1
A horizontal incision is made in a neck crease overlying the mass. Any fistula present is excised along with this incision. Subplatysmal flaps are then elevated over the cyst. The patient in Fig. 9 presented with a large lesion in close proximity to the inferior border of the mandible that necessitated a modified Blair incision for removal. Many times a smaller cyst in a more

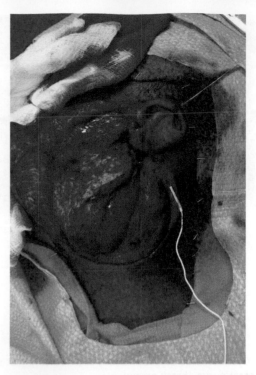

Fig. 9 Cyst visualized caudal to parotid gland and anterior to sternocleidomastoid muscle.

inferior position is easily accessed by a horizontal skin incision (see Fig. 9).

Step 2
At this point, a plane is usually easily developed around the cyst with gentle, blunt dissection (Fig. 10).

As dissection proceeds on the deep surface of the cyst, the surgeon must be aware of pharyngeal extensions that can

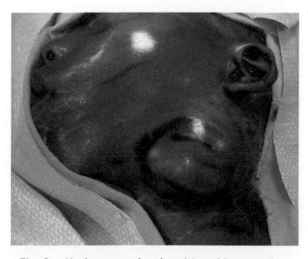

Fig. 8 Neck prepared and positioned in extension.

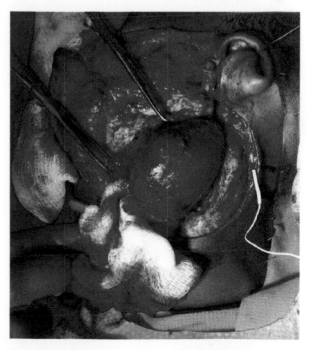

Fig. 10 Blunt dissection easily facilitates exposure and initial delivery of the cyst.

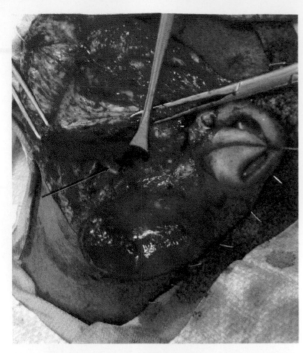

Fig. 11 Cyst tethered to deep tissues and coursing just superior to hypoglossal nerve (*black arrow*).

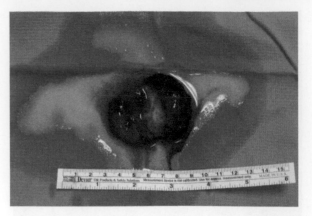

Fig. 12 Excised and bisected second brachial cleft cyst.

extend in close proximity to and in between the great vessels (Fig. 11). The hypoglossal nerve should be protected in this region as well. Blunt dissection along with judicious sharp dissection should allow the specimen to be removed entirely (Fig. 12).

Step 3

The incision is closed in layers starting with the subcutaneous tissues. Skin closure is obtained with 5-0 or 6-0 resorbable suture, skin adhesive and steristrips. Drain placement is typically not necessary.

Acknowledgments

The authors would like to thank Bruce B. Horswell MD, DDS, MS, for the wonderful series of photos on the Sistrunk procedure.

Further readings

Edwards SP. Pediatric malignant tumors of the head and neck. In: Bagheri SC, Bell RB, Khan HA, editors. Current therapy in oral and maxillofacial surgery. 1st edition. Saunders; 2011. p. 820–7.

Goins MR, Beasley MS. Pediatric neck masses. Oral Maxillofac Surg Clin North Am 2012;24:457–68.

Meier JD, Grimmer JF. Evaluation and management of neck masses in children. Am Fam Physician 2014;89:353–8.

Rosa PA, Hirsh DL, Dierks EJ. Congenital neck masses. Oral Maxillofac Surg Clin North Am 2008;20:339–52.

Neck Infections

Brent A. Feldt[a], David E. Webb, Maj, USAF, DC [b],*

KEYWORDS

- Neck infection • Abscess • Incision and drainage

KEY POINTS

- Understanding fascial planes and potential spaces within the neck is integral to determining routes of spread and mandatory when surgical intervention is necessary.
- Imaging is critical in the stable patient to determine the location and severity of infection as well as provide a guide when surgery is indicated.
- Pharmacologic treatment initially includes empiric broad-spectrum antibiotics against gram-positive, gram-negative, and anaerobic bacteria—later refined based on culture and sensitivity results.
- Surgical intervention is reserved for complicated or unstable patients, or those who are unresponsive to medical therapy.

Etiology

Most neck infections arise from extension from the upper aerodigestive tract. Dental infections are the most common etiology, followed by oropharyngeal infections.[1-5] Occasionally, cervical lymphadenitis can lead to neck abscess, especially in undertreated or inadequately treated infections. Surgical manipulation of the upper airway and pharynx can cause spread of oral and oropharyngeal flora to the deep neck spaces, thus potentiating infection. Other causes of neck infection include spread of infection from the paranasal sinuses, mastoid, and skin, as well as intravenous drug use, penetrating trauma, foreign bodies, malignant necrotic lymph nodes, and congenital cysts.

Anatomy

Regardless of the source of infection, understanding the fascial planes and potential spaces of the neck is key to diagnosis and management of neck infections (Figs. 1 and 2, Table 1). The fascial planes provide real and potential spaces (Table 2) for the containment and/or spread of infection from the neck to other parts of the body.[6]

Microbiology

Oropharyngeal flora, including aerobic and anaerobic bacteria, are the most common isolates seen in culture from neck

infections.[2,7-9] Common bacteria and fungi cultured from neck infections are shown in Box 1.

Treatment of these organisms requires an understanding of the responsiveness of the bacteria or fungus to antibiotics. For instance, atypical *Tuberculosis* and *Mycobacteria* often cause chronic fistulae if treated surgically, while *Staphylococcus* and *Streptococcus* species usually respond more favorably to surgery when required.

Diagnosis

History

Recent dental or surgical procedures in the upper aerodigestive tract; sick contacts; animal and insect exposures; intravenous drug use; trauma; and past medical history, including immunomodulating medicines, allergies, and human immunodeficiency virus (HIV)/acquired immunodeficiency syndrome (AIDS), hepatitis, diabetes, malignancy, and chemotherapy.

Symptoms include:

- Onset and duration of symptoms
- Pain, fever, and redness at the site
- Dysphagia, odynophagia, drooling, hot potato voice, trismus, otalgia

Physical examination should include

- Palpation of the neck mass, evaluating for tenderness, fluctuance, crepitus
- Nasal cavity, oral cavity, oropharynx, and ear canal visual inspection (see Fig. 3)
- Bimanual examination of the oral cavity and oropharynx and teeth
- Flexible fiberoptic awake upper airway evaluation

See Table 3 for findings associated with neck infections.

Disclosures: The views expressed in this material are those of the authors, and do not reflect the official policy or position of the US Government, the Department of Defense, or the Department of the Air Force.

[a] Department of Otolaryngology, David Grant USAF Medical Center, 101 Bodin Circle/SGCXA, Travis AFB, CA 94535, USA

[b] Department of Oral and Maxillofacial Surgery, David Grant USAF Medical Center, 101 Bodin Circle/SGDD, Travis AFB, CA 94535, USA

* Corresponding author.

E-mail address: david.webb.5@us.af.mil

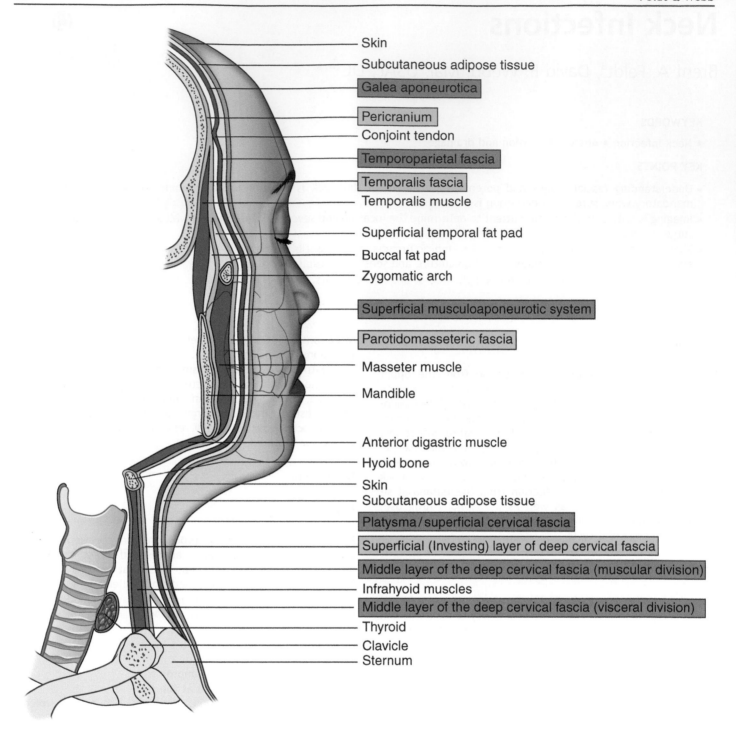

— Skin
— Subcutaneous adipose tissue
— Galea aponeurotica
— Pericranium
— Conjoint tendon
— Temporoparietal fascia
— Temporalis fascia
— Temporalis muscle
— Superficial temporal fat pad
— Buccal fat pad
— Zygomatic arch
— Superficial musculoaponeurotic system
— Parotidomasseteric fascia
— Masseter muscle
— Mandible
— Anterior digastric muscle
— Hyoid bone
— Skin
— Subcutaneous adipose tissue
— Platysma / superficial cervical fascia
— Superficial (Investing) layer of deep cervical fascia
— Middle layer of the deep cervical fascia (muscular division)
— Infrahyoid muscles
— Middle layer of the deep cervical fascia (visceral division)
— Thyroid
— Clavicle
— Sternum

Fig. 1 Anatomic representation of head and neck fascial planes. The superficial fascia (*maroon*) and deep fascia (superficial/investing layer, *blue*; middle layer, *purple*) of the head and neck are depicted. The white layer between the superficial and deep cervical fascia represents a potential space/surgical plane.

Laboratory evaluation should include

- Complete blood count:evaluate presence ofleukocytosis and pancytopenia
- Complete metabolic panel: evaluate for hyperglycemia, renal function, and hydration status

Imaging

Plain films have excellent clinical utility in neck infections. The retropharyngeal space and supraglottis are easily evaluated with lateral neck radiographs. A panoramic radiograph can help identify dental root abscesses not seen on physical examination.[6,8] Chest films should be obtained for stable patients with dyspnea, cough, and/or tachycardia to help rule out mediastinitis and pneumonia.

Computed tomography (CT) of the face and neck is critical in the stable patient for evaluation of neck infections. Physical examination alone often misidentifies or underestimates the extent of infection that can be seen on CT.[10–12] CT imaging can also help guide surgical planning by identifying involved spaces to be drained. Intravenous contrast should be used to

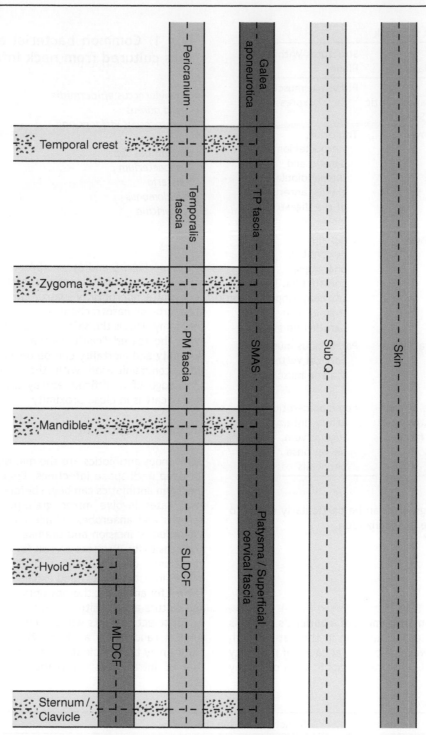

Fig. 2 Diagrammatic "roadmap" representation of head and neck fascial planes. Again the superficial fascia is maroon and the deep cervical fascia is blue and purple (SLDCF and MLDCF respectively). The superficial and deep fascia are continuous throughout the head and neck but change names at osseous "intersections." Note that only the muscular division of the MLDCF is represented. MLDCF, middle layer of the deep cervical fascia; PM, parotidomasseteric; SLCDF, superficial layer of the deep cervical fascia; SMAS, superficial musculoaponeurotic system; Sub Q, subcutaneous adipose tissue; TP, temporoparietal.

allow for optimal visualization of soft tissues and inflammation, unless patients have a known allergy to contrast or renal disease. Fluid-filled lymph nodes should be evaluated for malignancy, as both tonsillar and thyroid cancer can cause enlarged and necrotic lymphadenopathy mimicking abscess (Fig. 4).[13–15]

Magnetic resonance imaging is not routinely used for the diagnosis of neck infection. It can be helpful, however, if intracranial or neural extension is suspected.

Ultrasonography is becoming increasingly available in outpatient settings. The noninvasive nature, lack of radiation exposure, and low cost make it an attractive option for imaging

Table 1 Fascial layers of the neck

Fascial Plane	Common Name	Structures Within the Plane
Superficial cervical fascia	Superficial musculoaponeurotic system (SMAS)	Platysma, muscles of facial expression
Superficial layer of the deep cervical fascia	Investing layer	Trapezius, sternocleidomastoid, parotid and submandibular glands, anterior belly of the digastric, masseter
Middle layer of the deep cervical fascia	Visceral fascia	Strap muscles, buccinator, pharyngeal constrictors, larynx, trachea, esophagus, thyroid, and parathyroid glands
Deep layer of the Deep cervical fascia	Prevertebral fascia	Paraspinous muscles, cervical vertebrae, scalene muscle
Carotid sheath	Confluence of each layer of the deep cervical fascia	Common carotid artery, internal jugular vein, vagus nerve, ansa cervicalis

neck infections. Ultrasonography can be particularly useful to assist with needle drainage or localization.

Treatment

Airway management

As in any clinical scenario, management of a patient's airway is of highest priority. This is especially true in the patient with neck infection. Loss of airway is a potential cause of mortality in these patients.[16] Patients with radiographic signs of airway

Box 1. Common bacterial and fungal organisms cultured from neck infections

Staphylococcus epidermidis and aureus	*Haemophilus*
Streptococcus viridans and pyogenes	*Actinomyces*
Bacteroides spp.	*Tuberculosis*
Fusobacterium	*Mycobacteria*
Neisseria	*Bartonella henselae*
Pseudomonas	*Histoplasmosis*
Escherichia	*Coccidioides*

deviation (Figs. 5 and 6) or clinical findings (dyspnea, stridor, orthopnea, inability to control secretions) of impending airway necessitate fiberoptic visualization followed by awake fiberoptic oro- or nasotracheal intubation or cricothyrotomy/tracheotomy. This is the safest way to ensure a secure airway and avoid the feared "can't ventilate, can't intubate" scenerio. Morbidity and mortality can be decreased with early and constant communication with the anesthesia team, intimate knowledge of a difficult airway algorithm, and ensuring an airway cart is in close proximity.

Antibiotic treatment

Intravenous antibiotics are the mainstay of medical treatment for deep neck space infections. Empiric therapy with broad--spectrum antibiotics can begin before cultures return, because most cases involve mixed gram-positive and gram-negative aerobes and anaerobes. Fluids and/or tissue obtained from aspiration or incision and drainage should be sent for culture and sensitivity. Patients at risk for atypical infections, fungal infections, or methicillin-resistant *Staphylococcus aureus* (MRSA) infections may need expanded antibiotic coverage. See Table 4 for antibiotic therapy options based on clinical scenario and culture and sensitivity results.

For select patients without evidence of abscess or for poor surgical candidates, a 48- to 72-h trial of intravenous antibiotics may be sufficient treatment.[17–19] In stable children, a trial of intravenous antibiotics is recommended in almost

Table 2 Spaces of the neck

Space	Location	Structures Within the Space
Parapharyngeal	Suprahyoid neck	Prestyloid: fat, styloglossus, stylopharyngeus, lymph nodes, internal maxillary artery, deep lobe of parotid, V3 Poststyloid: carotid artery, jugular vein, sympathetic chain, CN IX, X, XI, XII
Submandibular and sublingual	Suprahyoid neck	Sublingual gland, Wharton' duct, submandibular gland, lymph nodes—teeth apices anterior to the mylohyoid (usually secon molar) involve the sublingual space
Peritonsillar	Suprahyoid neck	Loose connective tissue between palatine tonsil and superior constrictor muscle
Masticator	Face	Muscles of mastication, V3, buccal fat pad
Parotid	Face	Parotid gland, facial nerve, external carotid artery
Anterior visceral	Infrahyoid neck	Pharynx, esophagus, larynx, trachea, thyroid gland
Retropharyngeal space	Entire neck	Lymph nodes and connective tissue between the middle and deep layers of the deep cervical fascia
Danger/Prevertebral	Entire neck	Sympathetic chain, lymph nodes, extends from skull base to mediastinum and coccyx
Carotid	Entire neck	Carotid artery, internal jugular vein, vagus nerve, sympathetic chain, ansa cervicalis

Table 3 Findings associated with neck infections and possible etiology

Finding	Clinical Importance
Nasal cavity purulence	Retropharyngeal lymphadenopathy or swelling, foreign body
Uvular deviation	Peritonsillar or parapharyngeal space involvement, oropharyngeal malignancy (Fig. 3)
Teeth abscess	Odontogenic source, check for crepitus from gas-producing organisms
Posterior deflection of the tongue	Sublingual space involvement; "Ludwig angina" (Fig. 5)
Unilateral pharyngeal wall swelling with no erythema or fever	Parapharyngeal space tumor
Cranial neuropathy	Intracranial/neural extension
Hoarseness, dyspnea, stridor	Need to determine if airway is patent, midline, noninflamed or requires intubation or tracheostomy prior to imaging

all cases, as they have a higher likelihood of responding without surgical intervention.[20,21] Patients who fail to improve with intravenous antibiotics, repeat imaging should be obtained. Patients who respond well to intravenous antibiotics after 72 hours should be maintained on equivalent oral antibiotics for 10 to 14 days. Patients who require surgical intervention should have intravenous antibiotics for 48 to 72 hours postoperatively, and then a 10- 14-day course of an equivalent oral antibiotic.

Surgical treatment

Neck infections that are not responsive to medical management with intravenous antibiotics often require surgical drainage (Box 2).

The goals of surgical intervention are:

- Providing tissue and/or fluid for culture and sensitivity analysis
- Allowing for drainage and irrigation of isolated infected neck spaces and to prevent abscess reaccumulation

The first technique for drainage is needle aspiration (Fig. 7). This is usually best suited for small abscesses contained within cysts or superficial collections. It is often prudent to excise a cyst after aspiration and abatement of inflammation as fluid reaccumulation is probable.

Transoral drainage is often required for oral cavity, peritonsillar (Box 3, Figs. 8 and 9), and retropharyngeal abscesses,

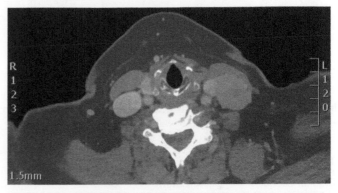

Fig. 4 CT scan of thyroid cancer metastatic to left cervical lymph nodes with signs of necrosis mimicking abscess.

as these areas are difficult to access through the neck. The retropharyngeal space abscess is first identified with needle aspiration, and then drained with an incision down through the submucosal layer. One of the oral cavity abscesses, Ludwig

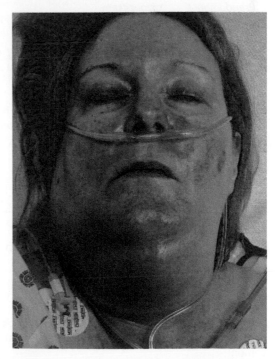

Fig. 5 Patient with Ludwig's angina. Ludwig's angina involves 5 spaces (bilateral submandibular, bilateral sublingual, and submental). Current mortality reduced to less than 10%.

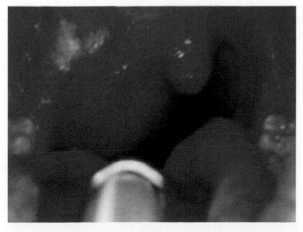

Fig. 3 Oropharyngeal exam in a patient with right peritonsillar abscess. (*Courtesy of* Dr Steven Maturo, San Antonio, Texas.)

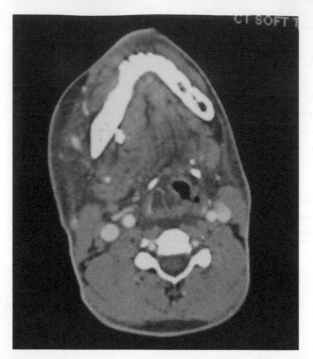

Fig. 6 Contrast-enhanced axial CT depicting neck infection resulting in airway deviation.

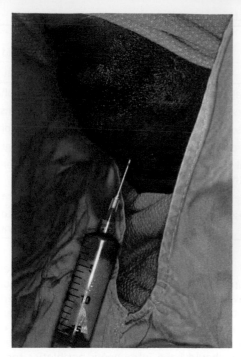

Fig. 7 Needle aspiration/sterile culture of superficial abscess.

Table 4 First-line antibiotics for neck infection treatment

Clinical Scenario	Antibiotic	Dose
Community-acquired infection with Gm+/ Gm−/anaerobic bacteria	Ampicillin-sulbactam	1.5—3 g intravenouysly (IV) every 6 h
	Clindamycin	600—900 mg IV every 8 h
Immunocompromised patients/nosocomial infection with MRSA and/or *Pseudomonas*	Ticarcillin-clavulanate	3 g IV every 6 h
	Piperacillin-tazobactam	3 g IV every 6 h
	Imipenem-cilastatin	500 mg IV every 6 h
	Ciprofloxacin	400 mg IV every 12 h
	Levofloxacin	750 mg IV every 24 h
	Clindamycin *plus*	600—900 mg IV every 8 h
	Vancomycin	1 g IV every 12 h if MRSA suspected
Necrotizing fasciitis	Ceftriaxone *plus*	2 g IV every 8 h
	Clindamycin *plus*	600—900 mg IV every 8 h
	Metronidazole	500 mg IV every 6 h

Box 2. Indications for surgical intervention in neck infection

1. Air—fluid level in the neck
2. Evidence of gas-producing organism
3. Abscess visualized in the fascial spaces of the neck
4. Threatened airway compromise from abscess or phlegmon
5. Failure to respond to 48 to 72 hours of empiric intravenous antibiotic therapy

angina, is best approached transcervically through the mylohyoid to help avoid airway embarrassment.

Neck spaces amenable to transcervical drainage can normally be approached by 1 of 3 incisions (Table 5).

Surgery proceeds with securing the airway with awake fiberoptic intubation or tracheotomy. The incision site is marked and injected with lidocaine with 1:100,000 epinephrine. Paralysis should be avoided to allow monitoring of cranial nerves.

The goal is to obtain sufficient access and drainage of the affected space to allow for irrigation and collection of fluid for culture and sensitivity. After incising through platysma, dissection into the affected space with a hemostat, Kitner followed by or blunt finger dissection allows for minimal damage to normal structures (Figs. 10 and 11). After obtaining tissue and/or fluid for culture, copious irrigation with normal

Box 3. Steps for transoral drainage of peritonsillar abscess

1. IV rehydration, 1 dose intravenous antibiotics and steroids
2. Small amount of topical anesthetic spray
3. Needle aspiration with 16- or 18-gauge needle and 5 to 10 cc syringe supero-lateral to the tonsil through the mucosa
4. If unsuccessful with aspiration, a 2 cm incision can be made through the mucosa and submucosa along the border of the tonsil into the abscess
5. Gentle spreading with hemostat will open the peritonsillar space and allow drainage of the abscess
6. Outpatient follow-up in 3 to 4 days to ensure abscess has not reaccumulated

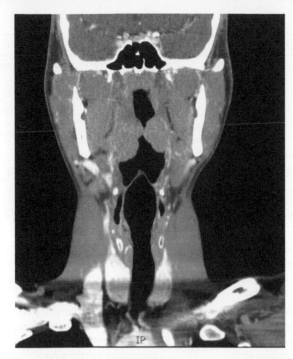

Fig. 8 Contrast enhanced coronal CT depicting right PTA shortly after elective third molar removal.

Table 5 Neck incisions for transcervical drainage

Incision	Space(s) Accessible
Preauricular modified Blair	Parotid, temporal
Horizontal neck incision in a natural skin crease	Masticator, parapharyngeal, pterygoid, submandibular, sublingual, prevertebral, retropharyngeal, carotid
Midline horizontal neck incision	Thyroid, trachea, esophagus, upper mediastinum, submandibular, submental

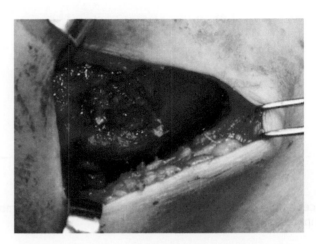

Fig. 10 Surgery for infected neck space. After incision and dissection through the platysma, infected and necrotic lymph node is identified.

saline should be undertaken. A Penrose drain can be brought out to the skin and sutured in place. Closure in layers is completed, and the patient is admitted for 48 to 72 hours of continued intravenous antibiotics while awaiting culture results.

Complications

Surgical complications are the same as for any neck surgery and include neurovascular injury including cranial neuropathy, paresthesia and paralysis or hemorrhage, reaccumulation of

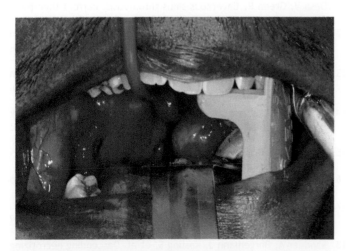

Fig. 9 Immediately after intraoral drainage of PTA—deferred quincy tonsillectomy.

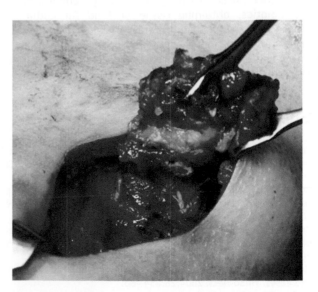

Fig. 11 Lymph node is dissected free from underlying structures. (*Courtesy of* Dr Steven Maturo, San Antonio, Texas.)

Table 6 Morbid complications associated with neck infections

Complication	Notes	Symptoms, Signs	Diagnosis and Management
Lemierre syndrome	• *Fusobacterium necrophorum* • Potentially fatal if untreated—mortality rate 5% even when treated	Fever, sore throat, lateral neck tenderness, trismus, septic emboli	CT with contrast showing internal jugular thrombosis Beta-lactamase resistant antibiotics +/− anticoagulation Surgery if unresponsive
Cavernous sinus thrombosis	• Often direct spread of *S. aureus* or *Streptococcus* from paranasal sinues • Mortality 30%–40%	"Picket-fence" fever, orbital pain, proptosis, decreased ocular motility, dilated pupil, sluggish pupil reflex	MRI with contrast Intensive care unit (ICU) care, broad spectrum IV antibiotics, anticoagulation
Carotid artery pseudoaneurysm	• Spread from retropharyngeal or parapharyngeal space	Pulsatile and tender neck mass, Horner syndrome, CN IX-XII palsy, hemorrhage	CT with contrast Surgical ligation of the carotid artery
Mediastinitis	• Mortality rate 30%–40%	Diffuse neck edema, dyspnea, pleuritic chest pain, tachycardia, hypoxia, mediastinal widening	CT scan with IV contrast Broad-spectrum IV antibiotics, transcervical or transthoracic drainage if unresponsive
Necrotizing fasciitis	• Often odontogenic origin in immunocompromised patient • Does not follow fascial planes • Mortality 20%–30%	Rapidly progressive cellulitis with pain out of proportion to exam, pitting neck edema, peau-d-orange skin appearance, subcutaneous crepitus	CT with contrast demonstrating tissue gas, liquefaction necrosis ICU care, treatment of immunocompromising conditions, broad-spectrum IV antibiotics, aggressive surgical debridement with frequent wash-outs, hyperbarics[22]

abscess, scarring, and orocutaneous fistula. Less common complications are shown in Table 6.

Summary

Neck infections are a common clinical finding in oral and maxillofacial practice. A focused history and physical examination are critical when determining infectious versus noninfectious etiology in the presence of neck swellings. Neck infections are a common clinical finding in oral and maxillofacial practice. Accurate diagnosis, prompt empiric intravenous antibiotics, obtaining tissue or fluid for culture and sensitivity and surgical intervention, when required, are essential for managing these infections. Complications are rare, but potentially life-threatening and require prompt intervention.

References

1. Boscolo-Rizzo P, Marchiori C, Montolli F, et al. Deep neck infections: a constant challenge. ORL J Otorhinolaryngol Relat Spec 2006;68:259–65.
2. Bottin R, Marioni G, Rinaldi R, et al. Deep neck infection: a present-day complications. A retrospective review of 83 cases (1998-2001). Eur Arch Otorhinolaryngol 2003;260:576–9.
3. Brook I. Microbiology and management of peritonsillar, retropharyngeal and parapharyngeal abscesses. J Oral Maxillofac Surg 2004;62:1545–50.
4. Huang TT, Liu TC, Chen PR, et al. Deep neck infection: analysis of 185 cases. Head Neck 2004;26:854–60.
5. Karkos PD, Asrani S, Karkos CD, et al. Lemierre's syndrome: a systematic review. Laryngoscope 2009;119(8):1552–9.
6. Marioni G, Rinaldi R, Staffieri C, et al. Deep neck infection with dental origin: analysis of 85 consecutive cases (2000-2006). Acta Otolaryngol 2008;128(2):201–6.
7. Gidley PW, Ghorayed BY, Stiernberg CW, et al. Contemporary management of deep neck space infections. Otolaryngol Head Neck Surg 1997;116:16.
8. Kinzer S, Pfeiffer J, Becker S, et al. Severe deep neck space infections and mediastinitis of odontogenic origin: clinical relevance and implications for diagnosis and treatment. Acta Otolaryngol 2009;129(1):62–70.
9. Parhiscar A, Har-El G. Deep neck abscess: a retrospective review of 210 cases. Ann Otol Rhinol Laryngol 2001;110:1051–4.
10. Crespo AN, Chone CT, Fonseca AS, et al. Clinical versus computed tomography evaluation in the diagnosis and management of deep neck infection. Sao Paulo Med J 2004;122:259–63.
11. Desa V, Green R. Cavernous sinus thrombosis: current therapy. J Oral Maxillofac Surg 2012;70(9):2085–91.
12. Elliott M, Yong S, Beckenham T, et al. Carotid artery occlusion in association with a retropharyngeal abscess. Int J Pediatr Otorhinolaryngol 2005;70:359–63.
13. Wang CP, Ko JY, Lou PJ, et al. Deep neck infection as the main initial presentation of primary head and neck cancer. J Laryngol Otol 2006;120:305–9.
14. Weber AL, Siciliano A. CT and MR imaging evaluation of neck infections with clinical correlations. Radiol Clin North Am 2000;38:941–68.
15. Vieira F, Allen SM, Stocks RM, et al. Deep neck infection. Otolaryngol Clin North Am 2008;41(3):459–83.
16. Karkos PD, Leong SC, Beer H, et al. Challenging airways in deep neck space infections. Am J Otolaryngol 2007;28:415–8.
17. Plaza Mayor G, Martinex-San Millan J, Martinez-Vidal A, et al. Is conservative treatment of deep neck space infections appropriate? Head Neck 2001;23:126–33.
18. Sandner A, Borgemann J, Kosling S, et al. Descending necrotizing mediastinitis: early detection and radical surgery are crucial. J Oral Maxillofac Surg 2007;65:794–800.

19. Tung-Yiu W, Jehn-Shyun H, Ching-Hung C, et al. Cervical necrotizing fasciitis of odontogenic origin: a report of 11 cases. J Oral Maxillofac Surg 2000;58:1347–52.

20. McClay JE, Murray AD, Booth T, et al. Intravenous antibiotic therapy for deep neck abscesses defined by computed tomography. Arch Otolaryngol Head Neck Surg 2003;129:1207–12.

21. Mora R, Jankowska B, Catrombone U, et al. Descending necrotizing mediastinitis: ten years' experience. Ear Nose Throat J 2004;83: 774–80.

22. Langford FP, Moon RE, Stolp BW, et al. Treatment of cervical necrotizing fasciitis with hyperbaric oxygen therapy. Otolaryngol Head Neck Surg 1995;112:274.

Hematopoietic Neck Lesions

Joshua E. Lubek, DDS, MD, FACS [a],*, Amro Shihabi, DMD, MD [a],
Laura A. Murphy, MD [b], Jason N. Berman, MD, FRCPC, FAAP [b,c,d,e,f]

KEYWORDS

- Lymphoma • Neck mass • Neck biopsy

KEY POINTS

- Lymphoma should be suspected in cases of painless unilateral enlarging neck mass.
- Lymphoma is generally categorized into both Hodgkin and Non-Hodgkin lymphoma.
- Open biopsy allows complete lymph node architectural and cytologic evaluation.
- The spinal accessory nerve can inadvertently be injured during supraclavicular lymph node biopsy.
- Current therapies for lymphoma include chemotherapy with/without local field radiotherapy.

Introduction

The head and neck contain approximately 300 lymph nodes. Both benign and malignant disease can cause enlargement of these cervical lymph nodes. Lymphoproliferative neck masses account for approximately 5% of all head and neck malignancies. Often these cancers present as painlessly enlarging unilateral neck masses. Lymphoma is generally classified into Hodgkin lymphoma (HL) or non-Hodgkin lymphoma (NHL). These disease categories are associated with specific histologic features, genetic profiles, and epidemiologic links. For example, the large, owl-eyed, multinucleated Reed-Sternberg cells are a hallmark of HL, but are not seen in NHL, in which significant morphologic heterogeneity is found between subtypes, including anaplastic large cell lymphoma and diffuse large B-cell lymphoma (DLBCL). Occurrence of NHL within extranodal sites within the head and neck (ie, Waldeyer's ring) is reported in approximately 30% of cases.[1,2] Accurate diagnosis is essential to identify the correct cytologic and biochemical markers and allow proper treatment to include both chemotherapy and radiotherapy.[3,4] This article focuses on presentation of lymphoma within the head and neck, various biopsy techniques, and a brief overview of current therapies in the management of lymphoma/hematopoietic malignancies.

Preoperative planning

The incidence of lymphoma has increased within the past decade. Lymphomas are generally categorized into 2 subtypes. HL, identified microscopically by the presence of Reed-Sternberg cells, often presents as a painless neck mass resulting from enlarged cervical lymph nodes. HL rarely involves the Waldeyer's ring or other head and neck extranodal sites. Often a single nodal chain is identified with spread to contiguous lymph nodes. In contrast, NHL has a higher incidence of extranodal presentation (30%) to include Waldeyer's ring, nasopharynx, and tongue base. Other sites within the head and neck include the oral cavity, paranasal sinuses, orbit, salivary glands, and thyroid gland. Lymphoma within the thyroid gland accounts for approximately 5% to 10% of all thyroid masses, often presenting with a rapidly enlarging thyroid mass, hoarseness, or dysphagia.[1,2,4]

Indolent lymphomas present as painless, slow-growing lymphadenopathy. Aggressive lymphoma presents as a rapidly growing mass with symptoms that depend on location, and can often invade vital structures.[1,4,5]

Constitutional or B symptoms (fever, weight loss, and night sweats) are more often found in HL and can help clinicians to differentiate a suspicious neck mass from the more common cause of metastatic squamous carcinoma. Decreased appetite, pruritic skin rash, and fatigue can also accompany these B symptoms.[4,5]

A neck mass suspected of lymphoma requires a thorough evaluation to include a complete history and physical examination, imaging, cytologic analysis (tissue biopsy), and bone marrow biopsy.

Imaging of the neck mass can include computed tomography (CT) scan, MRI, PET scan, and ultrasonography. In general, contrast-enhanced CT scan is the most common modality used to image a neck mass suspected to be lymphoma because it is necessary for tumor staging (Fig. 1). NHL nodes are often described as multiple small 1-cm to 2-cm nonnecrotic nodes

[a] Oral-Head Neck Surgery/Microvascular Surgery, Oncology Program, Greenebaum Cancer Center, University of Maryland, 650 West Baltimore Street, Room 1401, Baltimore, MD 21201, USA

[b] Department of Pediatrics, IWK Health Centre, Dalhousie University, 1348 Summer Street, Halifax, Nova Scotia B3H 4R2, Canada

[c] Clinician Investigator Program and Clinician Scientist Graduate Program, IWK Health Centre, Dalhousie University, 1348 Summer Street, Halifax, Nova Scotia B3H 4R2, Canada

[d] Division of Hematology/Oncology, IWK Health Centre, Dalhousie University, 1348 Summer Street, Halifax, Nova Scotia B3H 4R2, Canada

[e] Department of Microbiology and Immunology, IWK Health Centre, Dalhousie University, 1348 Summer Street, Halifax, Nova Scotia B3H 4R2, Canada

[f] Department of Pathology, IWK Health Centre, Dalhousie University, 1348 Summer Street, Halifax, Nova Scotia B3H 4R2, Canada

* Corresponding author.

E-mail address: jlubek@umaryland.edu

Atlas Oral Maxillofacial Surg Clin N Am 23 (2015) 31-37
1061-3315/15/$ - see front matter © 2015 Elsevier Inc. All rights reserved.
http://dx.doi.org/10.1016/j.cxom.2014.10.004

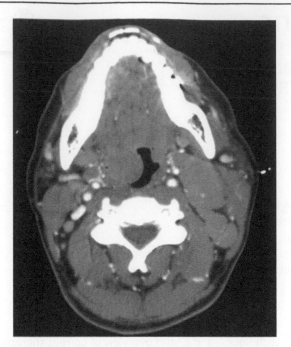

Fig. 1 CT scan of lymphoma involving both the tonsil and cervical lymph nodes. (*Courtesy of* Robert Morales, MD, Division of Neuroradiology, University of Maryland, Baltimore, MD.)

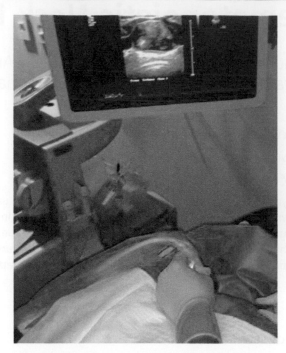

Fig. 2 Ultrasonography biopsy of suspected lymphoma within a thyroid mass. (*Courtesy of* Jade Wong MD, Department of Radiology, University of Maryland, Baltimore, MD.)

involving multiple nodal chains within the neck (occipital, retropharyngeal, levels II–V). There is often an enlarged dominant node that can range in size from 3 to 10 cm. Larger nodes with necrotic cores must be distinguished from squamous cell carcinomatous adenopathy, aggressive NHL, or lymphoma associated with acquired immunodeficiency syndrome. Nodal metastases from a distant primary, such as lung cancer or breast cancer, can be indistinguishable from NHL adenopathy on CT scan.[6–8]

The 2 main methods of establishing a tissue diagnosis include fine-needle aspiration biopsy (FNAB) and open biopsy technique. FNAB has the advantages of avoiding scars and minimizing risk to vital neck structures and bleeding risk. FNAB can often be combined with imaging, such as ultrasonography or CT scan, to improve accuracy of tissue sampling. Complete nodal architectural evaluation and subtype classification rates have been reported in various studies with 60% to 90% accuracy using ultrasonography-guided core biopsy (Figs. 2 and 3).[1,2,9–11]

Limitations of fine-needle aspiration biopsy

- Does not allow evaluation of nodal architecture
- Unable to provide histologic subtype because of inadequate sample
- Difficult to distinguish between reactive nodal hyperplasia and low-grade NHL
- Difficult to diagnose HL because of the required identification of Reed-Sternberg cells (not abundant within the tissue sample)
- Even when combined with flow cytometry, may be inadequate to diagnose disease

Open biopsy surgical technique

Despite the advantages of FNAB, open biopsy is still considered the gold standard for diagnosis of lymphoma because it

provides an adequate amount of tissue for diagnosis and cytologic architectural examination. Surgical risks and complications can be minimized with careful attention to detail by experienced surgeons. Open biopsy of a neck lymph node can be performed under general anesthesia or with local anesthetic techniques. Cervical plexus nerve blockade can be used to safely perform open biopsy under local anesthesia. Most surgeons prefer to perform open biopsy under general anesthesia for patient comfort, better control in the event of significant hemorrhage, better visibility, and avoidance of possible injury to vital anatomic structures caused by patient movements.[12]

Patient positioning

The patient is placed supine on the operating table and following induction of anesthesia the endotracheal tube is secured. Use of paralytic/muscle relaxant medications should be discussed with the anesthesia team preoperatively. Although not necessary in the identification of vital nerves (ie, marginal mandibular branch of the facial nerve, spinal accessory nerve), the ability to identify muscle twitching may help to alert the surgeon to the proximity of a named nerve and help avoid its inadvertent injury.

A shoulder roll is placed to allow neck extension and ease of access to the deeper structures of the neck if necessary. The patient is then prepped with an aseptic cleaning solution from the inferior border of the mandible to an area just inferior to the clavicles bilaterally. The patient is draped to allow exposure of cervical lymph nodes from levels I to V of the neck. Incisions are based on the specific lymph nodes to be biopsied. Careful evaluation of the preoperative imaging (ie, CT scan) helps to guide the surgeon as to the location of biopsy and vital anatomic structures within the region, and to select the lymph nodes with the easiest access.

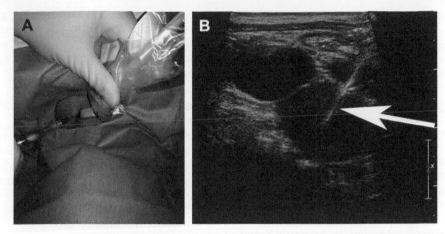

Fig. 3 Ultrasonography biopsy of suspected lymphoma within a neck mass. (*A*) Ultrasound guided needle biopsy of neck mass (*B*) *White arrow* demonstrates the needle passing into suspected lymphoma neck mass on ultrasound imaging. (*Courtesy of* Jade Wong, MD, Department of Radiology, University of Maryland, Baltimore, MD.)

Level IV/V and supraclavicular lymph node access

A low horizontal incision within a neck crease centered within level V/supraclavicular region is designed. The incision is made through the skin, subcutaneous tissue, and platysma muscle. The external jugular vein may be encountered and can either be retracted or ligated and divided with suture or metal clips. The posterior border of the sternocleidomastoid (SCM) muscle should be identified and retracted medially. The greater auricular nerve is identified exiting posteriorly from the sternocleidomastoid muscle and traveling superficially within the subcutaneous tissue toward the ear. This nerve is encountered if the incision is placed more superiorly for access to lymph nodes within the superior aspect of level V (apex of the triangle bounded between the SCM and trapezius muscles). Great care must be taken to identify the spinal accessory nerve within the posterior triangle (Figs. 4 and 5). This nerve often travels superficially as it enters the undersurface of the trapezius muscle. Blunt and sharp dissections are performed toward the lymph nodes with care to avoid injuring the various underlying structures. The SCM can be retracted medially and the inferior belly of the omohyoid muscle can be identified. The omohyoid muscle can either be retracted superiorly, inferiorly toward

the clavicle, or divided. Once deep to this muscle the internal jugular vein, brachial plexus, phrenic nerve, and carotid artery can be encountered. The transverse cervical vessels can be a landmark to alert the surgeon that the brachial plexus is in close proximity, bounded between the anterior and middle scalene muscles deep to these vessels. The surgeon must also be aware of the thoracic duct as it enters the deep venous system (internal jugular vein) on the left side of the neck or an accessory duct on the right neck. Lymphatic tissue should be ligated carefully or cauterized adequately to help avoid a chyle leak. The apex of the lung/pleura can be located in the supraclavicular fossa, increasing the risk of inadvertent lung injury and potential pneumothorax.[12]

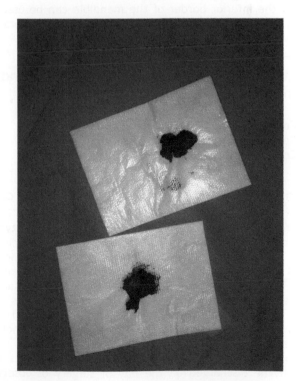

Fig. 5 Open biopsy of lymph node specimens. Tissue should be sent to pathology without placement in fixative solutions.

Fig. 4 Open biopsy within level V of the neck; the spinal accessory nerve can be visualized within the dissection (*black arrow*), and the external jugular vein identified anteriorly (*blue arrow*).

Level I to III lymph node access

A horizontal incision approximately 2 to 3 cm below the inferior border of the mandible within a neck crease allows both esthetic and functional access to these lymph nodes. Incision is carried through skin, subcutaneous tissue, and the platysma muscle. Subplatysmal flaps can be elevated superiorly and inferiorly. The external jugular vein and greater auricular nerve are visualized posteriorly superficial to the SCM. The SCM is then retracted laterally as dissection proceeds within the fibrolymphatic tissue deep to the SCM. The posterior belly of the digastric muscle should be identified superiorly. This muscle can be used as a landmark to identify the internal jugular vein deep to this muscle and the level II nodes. The spinal accessory nerve can be encountered in this region and meticulous attention to hemostasis and judicious use of cautery can help to avoid injury to cranial nerve (CN) XI. The hypoglossal nerve is usually identified at this level bounded between the internal jugular vein and the carotid artery. The nerve travels deep to the intermediate tendon of the digastric and course into the hyoglossus muscle and intrinsic muscles of the tongue. A plexus of veins can be encountered with this nerve and must be ligated carefully to avoid injury to the nerve. Level III lymph nodes can be identified along the internal jugular chain superior to the junction of the superior belly of the omohyoid as it crosses the SCM. Structures to be identified and preserved include the internal jugular vein, carotid artery, and vagus nerve. Access to lymph nodes within the submandibular triangle requires identification of the capsule of the submandibular gland and identification of the marginal mandibular branch of the facial nerve within the superficial layer of the deep cervical fascia within 2 cm of the inferior border of the mandible. The facial artery and vein can be encountered and ligated to gain access to these nodes. A Hayes-Martin maneuver involving ligation of the common facial vein at the level of the inferior border of the mandible can be used to retract the fascia superiorly, protecting the marginal branch of CN VII.[12]

Relationship of the spinal accessory nerve and the internal jugular vein at the skull base

- Courses anteriorly 70% to the vein
- Courses posteriorly 20% to 30% to the vein
- Courses through the vein approximately 1%

Wound closure and immediate postoperative care

Incisions can be closed in a layered fashion with the platysma reapproximated with a resorbable suture. Skin can be closed with a subcuticular suture technique, nonresorbable interrupted skin technique or staples. Depending on the extent of dissection, a suction drain or Penrose drain can be placed; however, this is often not necessary. Adhesive strips and topical skin ointments (eg, bacitracin) can be applied. Tissue for lymphoma diagnosis should be sent to anatomic pathology as a fresh specimen (do not place in formalin).

Pain medication should be prescribed and patients can generally be discharged on the day of surgery or observed overnight if concern for issues such as bleeding or hematoma is suspected. Standard perioperative-dose antibiotics should be prescribed but are not indicated for greater than 24 hours. Suture or staple removal is performed 5 to 7 days postoperatively. Once tissue diagnosis is established the patient continues with treatment under the care of the medical or radiation oncologist.

Caveats and potential complications

- Meticulous hemostasis with use of bipolar cautery helps to identify and protect vital structures such as the CNs
- Clear or milky-appearing fluid during lymph node removal within level IV/V should raise the suspicion of a thoracic duct or accessory duct injury
- Dissection posterior to the carotid artery can result in an ipsilateral Horner syndrome
- A suspected pneumothorax can be identified with a Valsalva maneuver by observing air bubbles arising within sterile saline at the surgical site
- Tissue for lymphoma diagnosis is sent to anatomic pathology in formalin rather than as a fresh specimen

Clinical results in the literature

Patients are categorized into one of 4 stages based on age, sites of involvement, presence and extent of bulky disease, and systemic symptoms.[4,5] Staging systems differ for children and adults, because children tend to have extranodal disease, whereas adults tend to have more restricted nodal involvement at the time of diagnosis. St. Jude staging is widely used in children with NHL (Table 1) and the Cotswold modified Ann Arbor staging is standard for childhood HL and adults with HL or NHL (Table 2).[5,13]

Each lymphoma generally behaves in a stereotypical fashion, which guides treatment strategies. Advances in

Table 1 St. Jude staging system for childhood NHL

Stage	Area of Involvement
I	Single tumor (extranodal) or anatomic area (nodal) excluding the mediastinum or abdomen
II	A single tumor (extranodal) with regional node involvement
	Two or more nodal areas on same side of diaphragm
	Two single (extranodal) tumors with or without regional node involvement on the same side of the diaphragm
	A resectable primary gastrointestinal tumor, with or without involvement of associated mesenteric nodes only
III	Two single tumors (extranodal) on opposite sides of the diaphragm
	Two or more nodal areas above and below the diaphragm
	All primary intrathoracic tumors
	All extensive intra-abdominal disease, unresectable
	All paraspinal or epidural tumors
IV	Any of the areas mentioned previously with initial CNS and/or bone marrow involvement

Abbreviation: CNS, central nervous system.

Table 2 Cotswold modified Ann Arbor staging system for lymphoma

Stage	Area of Involvement
I	Single lymph node group
II	Multiple lymph node groups on same side of diaphragm (or contiguous involvement of 1 extralymphatic organ or site 1 side of the diaphragm)
III	Multiple lymph node groups on both sides of diaphragm (which may be accompanied by splenic or extralymphatic organ involvement)
IV	Diffuse extranodal sites ± lymph node involvement
X	Bulk >10 cm
E	Extranodal extension or single, isolated site of extranodal disease
A	Without B symptoms
B	B symptoms: weight loss >10% of body weight in 6 mo; fever (>38°C [100.4°F] for 3 consecutive days), drenching night sweats

imaging have affected initial disease staging and treatment choices and are being used to assess interim response to treatment (discussed later). Gallium scanning provides additional information in identifying regions of active cell turnover, but the sensitivity and specificity of detection have been substantially improved with the recent incorporation of metabolic imaging in the form of PET scanning. These modalities have enhanced anatomic imaging by CT or MRI scan to effectively identify all sites of active disease.[7,8,12,14,15] Surgical resection is usually not undertaken in the management of HL, because these tumors are highly sensitive to chemotherapy and radiation and shrink substantially with treatment. The cornerstone of treatment of childhood NHL is chemotherapy (Table 3) because the disease may be widely disseminated at the time of diagnosis. Surgery is used to obtain diagnostic tissue, although occasionally tumors can be completely resected.[9,16] Chemotherapy is given to all patients with resected tumors to account for residual microscopic disease. In cases of relapse, high doses of chemotherapy and stem cell transplant are typically used.[3,5,17,18] Radiation is rarely used in NHL, unless the central nervous system or the testes are involved. Adult NHL is categorized as indolent or aggressive, and treatment regimens are based on subtype (Table 4). In general, treatment options for adult NHL include involved field radiotherapy (IFRT), combination chemotherapy, monoclonal antibody therapy, and/or autologous stem cell transplant.

General opinion with regard to the role of radiotherapy in both childhood and adult HL has been continually evolving.[17] Although cure can be achieved with radiation alone, long-term side effects, including risk of secondary malignancies, have resulted in the institution of more conformal radiation techniques (IFRT) (Fig. 6), reduced dosing, and combination treatment approaches with chemotherapy. These dual-therapy

Table 3 Treatment recommendations for pediatric NHL

Pediatric	B Cell	Lymphoblastic	Anaplastic
Early stage (I–II)	Resected 4–7 d of chemotherapy × 2 cycles Nonresected cytoreductive phase + 4 cycles chemotherapy	Chemotherapy (LSA2-L2 or BFM) divided into induction, consolidation, and maintenance therapy over 18 to 24 mo	Resected Cytoreductive phase + 3–6 cycles chemotherapy Nonresected Cytoreductive phase + 6 cycles chemotherapy
Advanced stage (III–IV)	Cytoreductive phase + 6–8 cycles of chemotherapy	CNS involvement Chemotherapy (LSA2-L2 or BFM) divided into induction, consolidation, and maintenance therapy + CRT No CNS involvement Chemotherapy (LSA2-L2 or BFM) divided into induction, consolidation, and maintenance therapy + HD MTX and intrathecal MTX	Doxorubicin, prednisone, and vincristine × 12 mo
Relapsed	Monoclonal antibodies Autologous or allogeneic stem cell transplant	Monoclonal antibodies Allogeneic stem cell transplant	Additional courses of standard chemotherapy + autologous or allogeneic stem cell transplant, novel biologic agents like crizotinib for ALK + tumors

Cytoreductive phase, Oncovin, prednisolone and fractionated cyclophosphamide.
LSA2-L2 and BFM: corticosteroids, vincristine, anthracyclines, L-asparaginase, cyclophosphamide, methotrexate, cytarabine, 6-mercaptopurine, 6-thioguaine. L-asparaginase and high dose methotrexate, given earlier in BFM.
Abbreviations: ALK+, anaplastic lymphoma kinase gene positive; BFM, Berlin-Frankfurt-Munster; CRT, cranial radiation technique; MTX, methotrexate.

Adapted from Hill B, Smith S. Cleveland Clinic for Continuing Education. Non-Hodgkin's and Hodgkin's Lymphoma. Available at: http://www.clevelandclinicmeded.com/medicalpubs/diseasemanagement/hematology-oncology/non-hodgkins-and-hodgkins-lymphoma/. Accessed October 15, 2014.

Table 4 Treatment recommendations for adult lymphoma

Adult	Indolent NHL	Aggressive NHL	HL
Early stage (I–II)	Observation	CHOP × 3 + IFRT	ABVD × 3 + IFRT
	IFRT	R-CHOP × 3	
Advanced stage (III–IV)	CHOP	R-CHOP × 6–8	ABVD × 6 + IFRT
	R-CHOP	CHOP or clinical trial for T cell	
	Observation		
Relapsed	Chemotherapy	Chemotherapy	Chemotherapy
	Autologous transplant	Autologous transplant	Autologous transplant
	Clinical trial	Clinical trial	Clinical trial

Indolent: follicular, chronic lymphocytic leukemia/small lymphocytic lymphoma, mantle cell.
Aggressive: diffuse large B cell, Burkitt.
Abbreviations: ABVD, doxorubicin (Adriamycin), bleomycin, vinblastine, and dacarbazine; CHOP, cyclophosphamide, hydroxydaunorubicin, vincristine (Oncovin), and prednisone; IFRT, involved field radiotherapy; R-CHOP, rituximab, cyclophosphamide, hydroxydaunorubicin, vincristine (Oncovin), and prednisone.

Adapted from Hill B, Smith S. Cleveland Clinic for Continuing Education. Non-Hodgkin's and Hodgkin's Lymphoma. Available at: http://www.clevelandclinicmeded.com/medicalpubs/diseasemanagement/hematology-oncology/non-hodgkins-and-hodgkins-lymphoma/. Accessed October 15, 2014.

strategies are intended to diminish both radiation-induced and chemotherapy-induced toxicities by using reduced doses of each modality. More recently, efforts to eliminate radiation have been undertaken by both adult and pediatric HL cooperative groups by using PET positivity after initial cycles of chemotherapy to determine which patients require radiotherapy. The addition of metabolic imaging is meant to facilitate the ability to distinguish scar tissue and fibrosis from active tumor cells following treatment. Although recent results from the Children Oncology Group intermediate-risk group study suggest that radiation can potentially be avoided for patients who have a complete response after 2 cycles of ABVE-PC (Adriamycin, bleomycin, vincristine, etoposide, prednisone, cyclophosphamide) chemotherapy, other pediatric and adult trials have shown improved outcomes for patients in whom radiotherapy was not omitted.[17,19] Results can be challenging to interpret because different trials include different disease stages, initial chemotherapy regimens differ, and overall salvage rates following recurrence are high, which influences overall survival.

At any given time, numerous clinical trials are enrolling patients with lymphoma. SWOG (Southwest Oncology Group) is the largest adult cancer clinical trial group in the United States. Major pediatric clinical trial groups include the Children's Oncology Group (COG) and St. Jude's Children's Research Hospital in the United States and the Berlin-Frankfurt-Munster (BFM) group in Europe. Clinical trials attempt to improve outcomes for higher risk lymphomas through the introduction of novel therapies, or attempt reductions in treatment intensity while maintaining positive outcomes for diseases associated with good survival and/or high salvage rates in the event of a recurrence. Positive results from recent trials that have included rituximab, which targets CD20 on B cells, have led to this becoming the standard therapy for many subtypes of B-cell NHL in children and adults. Histone deacetylase inhibitors, such as vorinostat and romidepsin, are being used as monotherapies or in combination to treat relapsed DLBCL and other B-cell lymphomas. Immunomodulation of the lymphoma microenvironment using drugs such as thalidomide derivatives like lenalidomide and pomalidomide is another evolving therapeutic strategy. Overall, clinical trials have led to extended event-free survival and improved quality of life for lymphoma survivors by reducing the frequency of long-term toxicities, such as heart disease, pulmonary symptoms, and impaired fertility.[18,20–23]

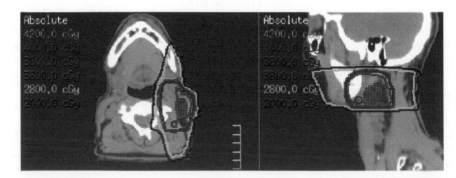

Fig. 6 CT scan marking the local area of treatment of a lymphoma mass within the neck (involved field radiotherapy). (*Courtesy of* Young Kwok, MD, Department of Radiation Oncology, University of Maryland, Baltimore, MD.)

Summary

HL and NHL represent a heterogeneous group of lymphoproliferative malignancies classified by the World Health Organization from phenotype (B/T lineage) and differentiation (precursor vs mature).[4,24] Lymphoma accounts for approximately 5% of all head and neck malignancy and is the most common diagnosis in young adults (20–40 years of age) who present with a unilateral enlarging neck mass. Lymphomas manifest with nodal or extranodal effects, and children are more likely to have extranodal involvement at the time of diagnosis.[1,2] The open lymph node biopsy technique is still considered the standard for establishing diagnosis of both HL and NHL, despite advances in ultrasonography-guided biopsy techniques. Childhood and adult HL are generally staged using the Cotswold modified Ann Arbor classification system. The Cotswold modified Ann Arbor system is also used to stage adult NHL, whereas the St. Jude staging classification is used for childhood NHL. Treatment of HL consists of chemotherapy and IFRT based on response. PET scanning is being used to determine which patients may benefit most from radiation therapy, although the ability to eliminate radiation in HL remains to be determined. Treatment of NHL varies by subtype, but generally includes combination chemotherapy, monoclonal antibody therapy, or stem cell transplant. The inclusion of rituximab has changed lymphoma outcomes, and as a result it is now part of the standard therapy in some childhood and adult B-lineage NHL.[18,21,22] Genetic profiling of subtypes of NHL are identifying driver mutations such as BCL2 in DLBCL, for which targeted biologic therapies are being developed and trialed.[3,20] Additional research efforts are being focused on altering the lymphoma microenvironment and epigenetic landscape with the promise of new effective antilymphoma agents.

References

1. Herd MK, Woods M, Anand A, et al. Lymphoma presenting in the neck: current concepts in diagnosis. Br J Oral Maxillofac Surg 2012; 50:309–13.
2. Urquhart A, Berg R. Hodgkin's and non-Hodgkin's lymphoma of the head and neck. Laryngoscope 2001;111:1565–9.
3. Bailey NG, Gross TG, Lim MS. Genomic basis of pediatric lymphomas. In: Dellaire G, Berman JN, Arceci R, editors. Cancer genomics: from bench to personalized medicine. 1st edition. Philadelphia: Elsevier; 2014. p. 342–57.
4. Campo E, Swerdlow SH, Harris NL, et al. The 2008 WHO classification of lymphoid neoplasms and beyond: evolving concepts and practical applications. Blood 2011;117:5019–32.
5. Reiter A, Ferrando A. Malignant lymphomas and lymphadenopathies. In: Orkin SH, Fisher DE, Look AT, et al, editors. Oncology of infancy and childhood. 1st edition. Philadelphia: Elsevier; 2009. p. 417–508.
6. Harnsberger HR, Bragg DG, Osborn AG, et al. Non-Hodgkin lymphoma of the head and neck: CT evaluation of nodal and extranodal sites. AJR Am J Roentgenol 1987;8:673–9.
7. Weber AL, Rahemtullah A, Ferry JA. Hodgkin and non-Hodgkin lymphoma of the head and neck: clinical pathologic and imaging evaluation. Neuroimaging Clin N Am 2003;13:371–92.
8. Harnsberger HR, Wiggins RH, Hudgins PA, et al. Diagnostic imaging head and neck. 3rd edition. Salt Lake City (UT): Amirsys; 2006.
9. Morris-Stiff G, Cheang P, Key S, et al. Does the surgeon still have a role to play in the diagnosis and management of lymphomas? World J Surg Oncol 2008;6:13–6.
10. Cannon CR, Richardson D. Value of flow cytometry with fine needle aspiration biopsy in patients with head and neck lymphoma. Otolaryngol Head Neck Surg 2000;123:696–9.
11. Lister TA, Crowther D, Sutcliffe SB, et al. Report of a committee convened to discuss the evaluation and staging of patients with Hodgkin's disease: Cotswolds meeting. J Clin Oncol 1989;7(11): 1630–6.
12. Medina JE, Lore JM. The neck. In: Lore JM, Medina JE, editors. An atlas of head and neck surgery. 4th edition. Philadelphia: Elsevier; 2005. p. 980.
13. Armitage JO. Staging non-Hodgkin lymphoma. CA Cancer J Clin 2005;55:368–76.
14. Cheson BD. New staging and response criteria for non-Hodgkin lymphoma and Hodgkin lymphoma. Radiol Clin North Am 2008;46: 213–23. vii.
15. Burke C, Thomas R, Inglis C, et al. Ultrasound guided core biopsy in the diagnosis of lymphoma of the head and neck. A 9 year experience. Br J Radiol 2011;84:727–32.
16. Coran GA, Caldamone AN, Adzick S, et al. Hodgkin and non-Hodgkin lymphoma. In: Ehrlich P, editor. Pediatric surgery. Philadelphia: Saunders; 2012. p. 517–28.
17. Johnson PW. Management of early-stage Hodgkin lymphoma: is there still a role for radiation? Hematology Am Soc Hematol Educ Program 2013;2013:400–5.
18. Coiffier B. Rituximab therapy in malignant lymphoma. Oncogene 2007;26:3603–13.
19. Friedman DL, Chen L, Wolden S, et al. Dose-intensive response based chemotherapy and radiation therapy for children and adolescents with newly diagnosed intermediate risk hodgkin lymphoma: a report from the children's oncology group study AHOD0031. J Clin Oncol 2014;32:3651–8.
20. Ott G, Rosenwald A, Campo E. Understanding MYC-driven aggressive B-cell lymphomas: pathogenesis and classification. Hematology Am Soc Hematol Educ Program 2013;2013:575–83.
21. Mounier N, Briere J, Gisselbrecht C, et al. Rituximab plus CHOP (R-CHOP) overcomes bcl-2–associated resistance to chemotherapy in elderly patients with diffuse large B-cell lymphoma (DLBCL). Blood 2003;101:4279–84.
22. Yustein JT, Dang CV. Biology and treatment of Burkitt's lymphoma. Curr Opin Hematol 2007;14:375–81.
23. Li S, Gill N, Lentzsch S. Recent advances of IMiDs in cancer therapy. Curr Opin Oncol 2010;22:579–85.
24. Swerdlow SH, Campo E, Harris NL, et al. WHO classification of tumors of hematopoietic and lymphoid tissues, 4th edition. Lyon (France): International Agency for Research on Cancer (IARC); 2008.

Procedure/Technique

Endocrine Tumors of the Neck

Rui Fernandes, MD, DMD [a],*, Mark Allen Miller, MD, DMD [b],
Anthony Morlandt, DDS, MD [c]

KEYWORDS

- Thyroid • Parathyroid • Multinodular goiter • Graves disease • Papillary carcinoma of thyroid • Parathyroid adenoma
- Recurrent laryngeal nerve • Hypocalcemia

KEY POINTS

- Routine use of computed tomography or MRI is not recommended in the work-up of cervical thyroid disease, but may be useful in evaluation of substernal thyroid to estimate the need for sternotomy.
- Preoperative laryngoscopy is indicated for patients presenting voice changes, neurosensory disturbances, and for reoperative surgery.
- Diagnostic ultrasonography of the thyroid should be ordered in all patients with a suspected malignancy, nodule, or multinodular goiter; incidental thyroid or parathyroid masses noted on routine imaging may warrant further investigation with fine-needle aspiration cytology.
- Because thyroidectomy and parathyroidectomy are typically elective procedures, potentially confounding medical comorbidities are addressed before surgery.
- Direct intraoperative visualization of the recurrent laryngeal nerve is the standard of care and decreases the incidence of injury to the nerve.
- The need for thyroid hormone supplementation depends on the postoperative diagnosis and should be coordinated with the consulted/referring endocrinologist.
- There is a risk for developing transient or permanent postoperative hypoparathyroidism after thyroid surgery.
- Routine elective calcium supplementation following thyroidectomy has been shown to prevent symptoms of hypocalcemia.

Introduction

Thyroidectomy and parathyroidectomy were once associated with significant surgical morbidity but are now the most common ablative tumor procedures performed by head and neck surgeons.[1] The indications for thyroidectomy vary by surgeon and institution, but are performed for a variety of benign and malignant conditions.

Pertinent anatomy and physiology

Understanding the embryonic development of the thyroid and parathyroid glands, the recurrent laryngeal nerve (RLN), and the external branch of the superior laryngeal nerve (EBSLN) is paramount to successful endocrine surgery (Fig. 1). The thyroid gland arises from 2 sources: the neural crest and the primitive pharynx endoderm. The main body of the thyroid gland is derived from epithelial cells of the primitive pharynx endoderm, later undergoing differentiation into discrete follicles that produce and secrete thyroid hormone. The parafollicular C cells, responsible for calcitonin production, develop from the neural crest. The thyroglossal duct may persist at any level from the foramen cecum to the pyramidal lobe of the thyroid gland. The parathyroid glands arise from the third and fourth pharyngeal pouches early during embryologic development, and can occupy variable positions along the neck and mediastinum. The RLN recurs around the lowest extant aortic arch in the mediastinum, the fourth arch on the right, which persists as the subclavian artery, and the sixth arch on the left, which remains as the ligamentum arteriosum (Fig. 2).

The thyroid gland weighs about 20 to 25 g and is composed of 2 lateral lobes connected by the isthmus. It is invested in a true capsule and lies anterior to the cricoid cartilage and trachea, and inferior to the thyroid cartilage. The isthmus of the thyroid overlies the second and third tracheal rings. The gland is enclosed within the pretracheal fascia, and is fixed posteriorly by a condensation of this fascia known as the Berry ligament to the trachea and the laryngopharynx. The gland has a fibrous outer capsule, and is overlaid anteriorly by the infrahyoid (strap) muscles.

[a] University of Florida College of Medicine-Jacksonville, 653-1 West 8th Street, LRC Building, 2nd Floor, Jacksonville, FL 32209, USA
[b] Oral & Maxillofacial Surgery, University of Florida College of Medicine-Jacksonville, Jacksonville, FL, USA
[c] Oral Oncology and Microvascular Surgery, Oral and Maxillofacial Surgery, University of Alabama at Birmingham, Birmingham, AL, USA
* Corresponding author.
E-mail address: rui.fernandes@jax.ufl.edu

Atlas Oral Maxillofacial Surg Clin N Am 23 (2015) 39–47
1061-3315/15/$ - see front matter © 2015 Elsevier Inc. All rights reserved.
http://dx.doi.org/10.1016/j.cxom.2014.10.007

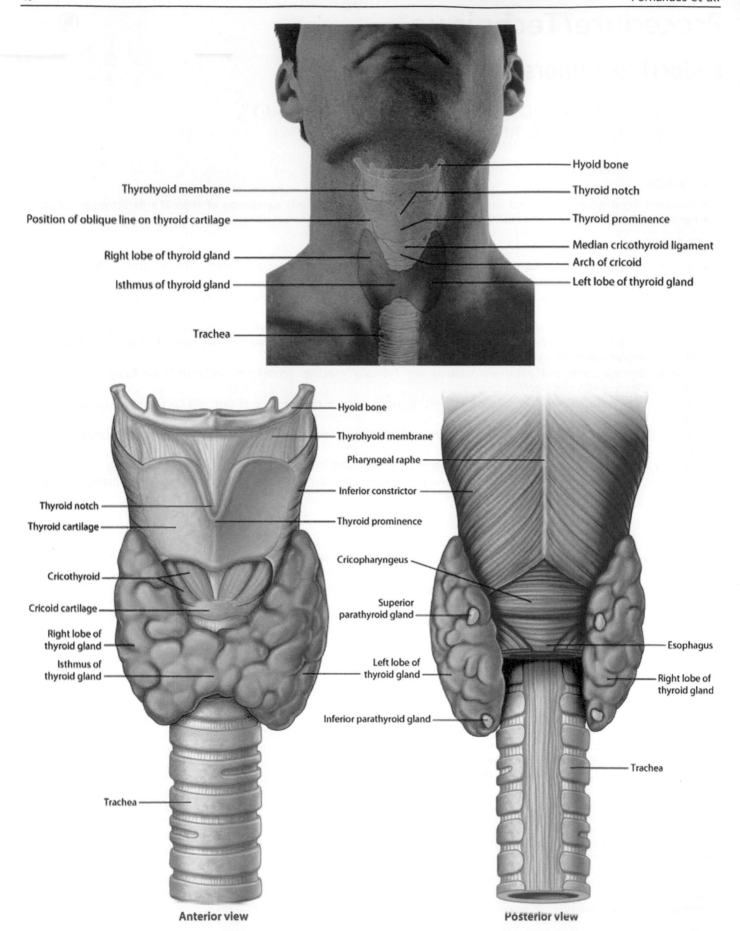

Fig. 1   Normal thyroid and parathyroid gland anatomy. (*From* Drake RL, Vogl AW, Mitchell AWM. Gray's atlas of anatomy. 2nd edition. Philadelphia: Churchill Livingstone, an imprint of Elsevier, 2015; with permission.)

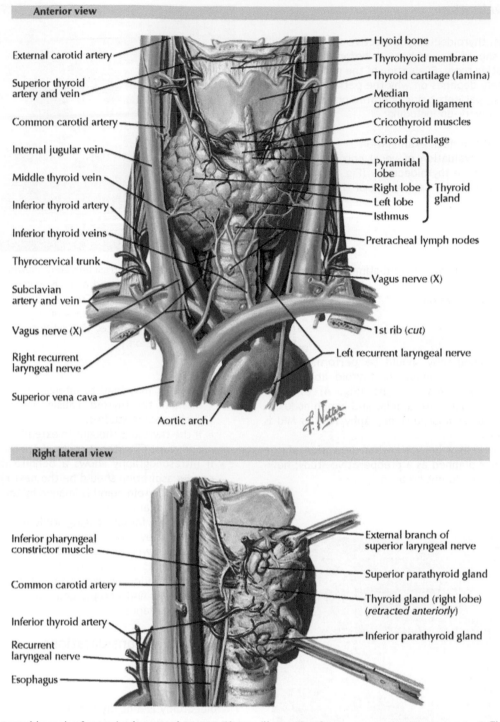

Anterior view

External carotid artery

Superior thyroid artery and vein

Common carotid artery

Internal jugular vein

Middle thyroid vein

Inferior thyroid artery

Inferior thyroid veins

Thyrocervical trunk

Subclavian artery and vein

Vagus nerve (X)

Right recurrent laryngeal nerve

Superior vena cava

Aortic arch

Hyoid bone

Thyrohyoid membrane

Thyroid cartilage (lamina)

Median cricothyroid ligament

Cricothyroid muscles

Cricoid cartilage

Pyramidal lobe

Right lobe — Thyroid gland

Left lobe

Isthmus

Pretracheal lymph nodes

Vagus nerve (X)

1st rib (cut)

Left recurrent laryngeal nerve

Right lateral view

Inferior pharyngeal constrictor muscle

Common carotid artery

Inferior thyroid artery

Recurrent laryngeal nerve

Esophagus

External branch of superior laryngeal nerve

Superior parathyroid gland

Thyroid gland (right lobe) (retracted anteriorly)

Inferior parathyroid gland

Fig. 2   RLN and external branch of superior laryngeal nerve. (Netter illustration from www.netterimages.com. © Elsevier Inc. All rights reserved.)

Two branches of the vagus nerve are intimately associated with the thyroid gland and are at risk of injury during thyroidectomy surgery: the RLN and EBSLN. The RLN courses in the tracheoesophageal groove toward its insertion into the cricothyroid muscle. It follows an oblique course on the right side and a more vertical orientation on the left. The superior and inferior parathyroid glands are found near the middle and lower poles of the thyroid lobes respectively.

The thyroid receives blood supply from the superior thyroid artery, a branch of the external carotid, and the inferior thyroid artery, which arises from the thyrocervical trunk. These arterial branches enter the gland beneath the pretracheal fascia and enter the underlying parenchyma.

Venous drainage is achieved by 3 veins: the superior and middle thyroid veins, which drain directly into the internal jugular vein; and the inferior thyroid vein, which drains into the brachiocephalic (innominate) vein.

Preoperative evaluation

With few exceptions, thyroidectomy is elective surgery and all medical concerns should be addressed before taking the patient to the operating room. Evaluation of the patient before thyroid surgery largely depends on why the patient needs the operation. In general, patients being operated on for a thyroid nodule should have a work-up including:

- A complete head and neck examination
- Laryngoscopy for evaluation of vocal cord mobility, especially in reoperative thyroidectomy (Fig. 3)
- Fine-needle aspiration for assessment of thyroid nodules

Laboratory testing

- Serum calcium level
- Thyroid function including thyroid-stimulating hormone and free tyroxine (T4)
- Endocrinologist consultation

Imaging studies

- Diagnostic ultrasonography should be performed in all patients with a thyroid nodule or thyroid abnormality detected by another imaging type (Fig. 4) to allow assessment of the contralateral lobe and lymph nodes.
- The routine use of computed tomography (CT) or MRI is not recommended.
  - CT of the neck may be used when resection of the thyroid gland is planned as a preoperative study; however, contrast should not be used.

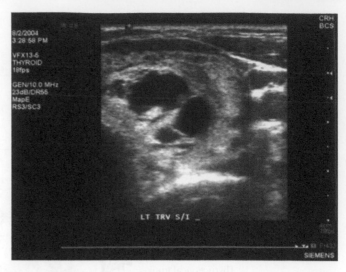

Fig. 4 Preoperative ultrasonography showing a large left thyroid colloid nodule that has solid and cystic components. This nodule was treated by lobectomy. (*From* Townsend CM, Beauchamp RD, Evers BM, et al. Sabiston textbook of surgery: the biological basis of modern surgical practice. 18th edition. Philadelphia: Saunders; 2008; with permission.)

  - Contrast may lead to intense and prolonged enhancement of the thyroid, causing interference with radioactive iodine studies.
  - If the thyroid is thought to extend substernal, then neck and chest CT without contrast are useful for evaluation.
- If ultrasonography shows a definite mass, then a fine-needle aspiration should be the next clinical step.
- The parathyroid gland is imaged by the Sestamibi nuclear medicine scan.
  - Preferred initial imaging study for parathyroid disease marked by high serum parathyroid hormone (PTH) levels as well as increased serum calcium levels.
  - In patients with recurrent or persisting hyperparathyroidism following exploration of the neck, MRI has been useful to find ectopic and nonectopic abnormal parathyroid glands.

Perioperative considerations

Antibiotics

Thyroidectomy is a highly vascular, clean procedure with very low postoperative infection rates.[2] A perioperative antibiotic, such as cefazolin, can be used in immunocompromised patients or in patients with multiple medical comorbidities that would result in an increase in risk for infection.

Intraoperative neuromonitoring

Iatrogenic injury to the RLN is a major concern during thyroid surgery.[3] The standard of care is direct visualization of the RLN, which decreases the incidence of injury.[4] Intraoperative neuromonitoring is often used to aid in identification and dissection of the RLN, and postprocedure testing of laryngeal function.[5] It is considered to be most useful in reoperative situations. The patient is intubated with a specialized laryngeal monitoring tube. Electrodes are placed in contact with

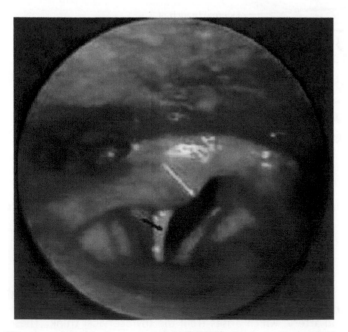

Fig. 3 Videolaryngoscopy of unilateral vocal cord paralysis. Right vocal cord (*black arrow*) is lateralized and flaccid, and the arytenoid (*white arrow*) is anteriorly located. (*From* Su WF, Hsu YD, Chen HC, et al. Laryngeal reinnervation by ansa cervicalis nerve implantation for unilateral vocal cord paralysis in humans. J Am Coll Surg 2007;204(1):64–72; with permission.)

the vocalis muscles bilaterally, and electromyography is monitored intraoperatively. It is imperative that only short-acting muscle relaxants such as succinylcholine are used during induction.

Surgical approach and procedure

Thyroid lobectomy and isthmusectomy

Positioning
The patient is prepped and draped in the supine position over a shoulder roll.[6] Extension of the neck promotes visualization of the surgical field and optimizes delivery of the specimen.

Surgical approach
A transverse incision is designed in a natural skin crease, 3 to 4 cm above the sternal notch. The incision ideally is marked preoperatively with the patient seated upright (Fig. 5). In young female patients, eventual inferior displacement of the scar with gravity and age will result in the scar being well hidden in the shadow of the sternal notch.

Skin and subcutaneous tissues are incised. Subplatysmal flaps are raised superiorly to the hyoid bone and inferiorly to the sternal notch and clavicles. Care is taken to avoid injury to the anterior jugular veins in the subplatysmal plane. These vessels may be controlled with 2-0 silk ties or vascular clips to minimize troublesome bleeding. Next, a Mahorner retractor or 2-0 silk tie-back sutures are applied to the skin flaps to enhance visualization.

Exposure of thyroid capsule
The linea alba is divided vertically and the strap muscles separated in the midline, exposing the thyroid isthmus and pyramidal lobe (when present). At this point, delivery of the thyroid lobe consists of identification and ligation of 3 vessel systems: superior thyroid artery and vein, middle thyroid vein, and inferior thyroid artery and vein. A capsular dissection is maintained throughout the procedure to minimize injury to the RLN, EBSLN, and parathyroid glands (Fig. 6).

Mobilization of gland and identification of recurrent laryngeal nerve
Next, the middle thyroid vein is identified and suture ligated as close to the capsule as possible, which permits further medial retraction of the gland over the trachea, separating the tracheoesophageal groove and allowing identification of the RLN. The nerve is exposed by gently spreading in the direction of its course to avoid inadvertent neuropraxia. Superficial branches of the inferior thyroid vein may be safely ligated and divided in this area; however, care must be taken to avoid injury to the underlying nerve (if the RLN is not identified at this point, a nonrecurrent laryngeal nerve may be suspected).

Delivery of inferior pole
Following identification and preservation of the RLN, the inferior pole may be mobilized with Kittner sponges, retracted superomedially, and the inferior thyroid artery suture ligated and divided. During this maneuver the inferior parathyroid gland is typically identified by its peanut-butter color. The vascular supply to the parathyroid gland may be preserved by ligating arterial branches to the thyroid gland as close to the capsule as possible. If the parathyroid becomes ischemic during elevation of the thyroid gland, it may be explanted, minced into 1 mm cubes, and reimplanted into the sternocleidomastoid or brachioradialis muscle.

Delivery of superior pole
A Goelet bull nose retractor is used to retract the sternothyroid and sternohyoid muscles laterally, and an appendiceal retractor superiorly exposes the superior pole (in the case of advanced multinodular goiter with a large gland, division of a few fibers of the sternothyroid muscle eases visualization of the upper pole; the muscle may be repaired primarily at the conclusion of the case). Using 2 Kittner sponges, the upper pole is retracted laterally, and the superior thyroid veins are ligated and divided in a stepwise fashion. The avascular plane between

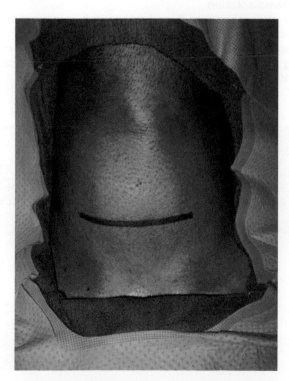

Fig. 5 Incision is marked overlying the cricoid cartilage, 2 to 3 fingerbreadths above the sternal notch.

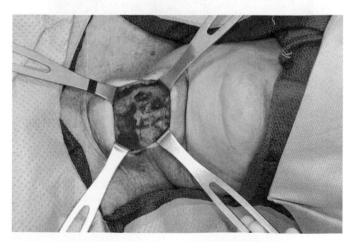

Fig. 6 Subplatysmal flaps are elevated, exposing the thyroid capsule.

the cricothyroid muscle and gland is developed bluntly using a Kittner sponge. The superior thyroid artery is then suture ligated and divided.

Division of the fibers of the posterior suspensory (Berry) ligament permits medial retraction of the gland over the anterior surface of the trachea (Fig. 7). The excised lobe, pyramidal lobe, and isthmus are delivered entirely. If a total thyroidectomy is performed, the identical procedure is performed for the contralateral lobe.

Wound closure

The wound is irrigated and approximated in layers over a closed suction drain, taking care to avoid excessively tight closure of the strap muscles. A running subcuticular closure is used to optimize esthetics.

Parathyroidectomy

Removal of select parathyroid glands (targeted parathyroidectomy) is indicated in adenomatous disease or carcinoma. Secondary hyperparathyroidism caused by renal dysfunction or hyperplasia resulting from MEN (multiple endocrine neoplasia) syndrome is typically treated surgically by subtotal parathyroidectomy or with total parathyroidectomy and autotransplantation of 50% of 1 gland into the sternocleidomastoid or brachioradialis muscle.

Surgical approach

Patient positioning, surgical incision, and approach to the thyroid gland are identical to thyroidectomy as described earlier. On mobilization of the inferior pole of the thyroid gland and identification of the RLN, the inferior parathyroid gland is identified close to the thyroid gland. Preoperative Sestamibi imaging may be useful in identifying prevertebral, retroesophageal, or mediastinal parathyroid glands (Fig. 8).

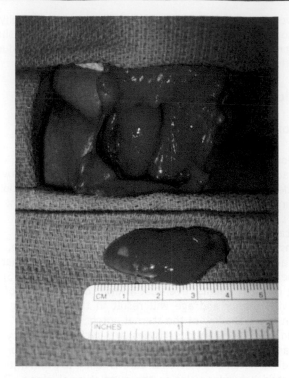

Fig. 8   Excised right inferior parathyroid adenoma.

Assessment of gland excision

Approximately 10 minutes after the adenoma is excised, a rapid intraoperative PTH is drawn from the patient's serum. A decrease of 50% from preoperative PTH levels is expected. As an alternative, the excised adenoma may be placed in saline; if the lesion floats it is likely adipose and not parathyroid tissue (Fig. 9).

Autotransplantation

Replantation of 50% of 1 excised gland is recommended to minimize hypocalcemia postoperatively. The parathyroid gland is minced into cubes of 1 to 2 mm, placed into the brachioradialis muscle, and the wound closed with absorbable suture (Fig. 10).

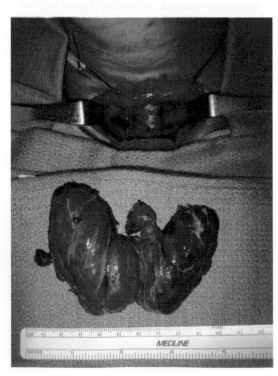

Fig. 7   Specimen delivered from the anterior surface of the trachea.

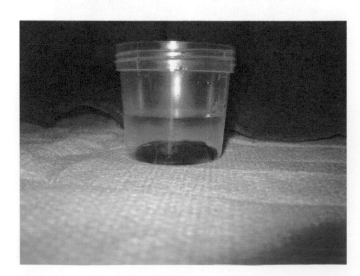

Fig. 9   Excised parathyroid tissue is expected to sink in normal saline.

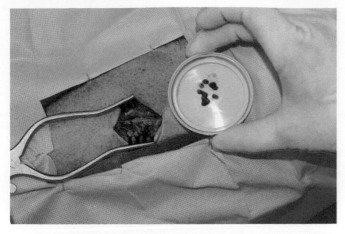

Fig. 10 The excised parathyroid gland is minced and placed into the brachioradialis muscle.

The cervical wound is irrigated and closed in similar fashion to the thyroidectomy procedure.

Case report: metastatic papillary carcinoma of the thyroid presenting as lateral neck mass

A 31-year-old man with no prior medical history presented with a slowly growing, nonpainful mass in left level II. Preoperative Doppler imaging was consistent with a nonvascular lesion, despite splaying of the carotid bifurcation noted on CT (suggestive of carotid body tumor) (Figs. 11 and 12).

The lesion was evaluated using fine-needle aspiration cytology, which was diagnostic. Open excision revealed metastatic papillary thyroid carcinoma (Figs. 13 and 14).

Definitive treatment involved bilateral neck dissection (I–V), central compartment dissection, and total thyroidectomy (Figs. 15–17).

Caveats/Potential complications

- Neck scar with hypertrophy or keloid formation
- Parathyroid injury or inadvertent removal, with resultant hypocalcemia

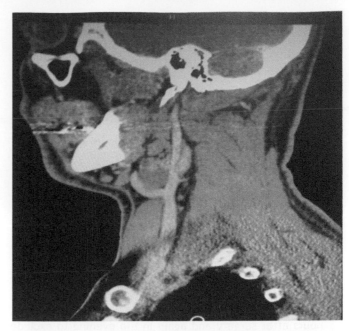

Fig. 12 Left-sided neck mass in 31-year-old patient.

- RLN injury with vocal cord fixation, increased risk of aspiration, and/or dysphagia
- EBSLN voice change caused by cricothyroid muscle paralysis
- Postoperative hematoma

Immediate postoperative care

- Patients may be observed overnight for the management of nausea, pain, and hypocalcemia.

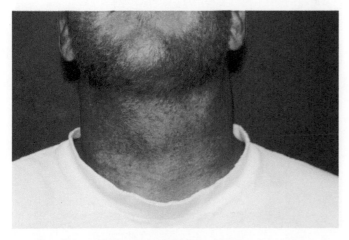

Fig. 11 Left-sided neck mass in 31-year-old patient.

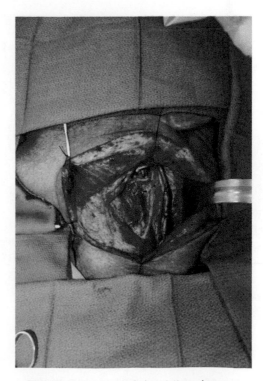

Fig. 13 Excised left level II neck mass.

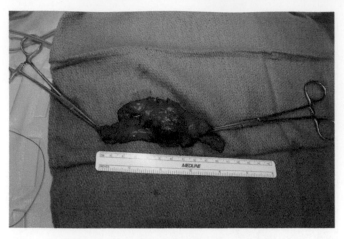

Fig. 14 Excised left level II neck mass.

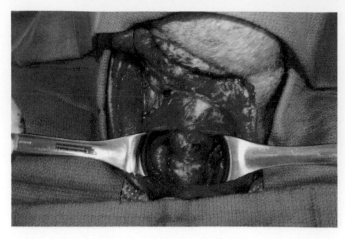

Fig. 16 Completed ND (VI).

- Patients must have a postoperative examination several hours after surgery and again in the evening to exclude the development of a hematoma. Postoperative hematomas can be life threatening secondary to airway compromise; immediate treatment is warranted. Most hematomas are associated with postoperative nausea and vomiting, or with violent coughing against the endotracheal tube on emergence from anesthesia.[7] Discussing deep extubation with the anesthesiologist is recommended.
- Hypocalcemia may be transient or permanent following thyroidectomy. The routine use of oral calcium and vitamin D has been shown to decrease the need for

intravenous calcium and development of hypocalcemic symptoms, allowing early and safer discharge.[8]
- Patients undergoing total parathyroidectomy are at risk of developing hungry bone syndrome; a prolonged, symptomatic hypocalcemia with hypomagnesemia and hypophosphatemia. Intravenous calcium infusion with oral supplementation is administered until the serum calcium levels are corrected.
- The recommendations for thyroid hormone supplementation depend on the final postoperative diagnosis and should be based on the recommendations of the consulting endocrinologist.

Rehabilitation and recovery

A postoperative follow up visit in 1 to 2 weeks is scheduled to evaluate the patient for voice changes as well as hypocalcemic symptoms. Surgical pathology findings are reviewed with the patient and additional therapies (thyroid hormone supplementation, calcium supplementation, and so forth) are initiated.

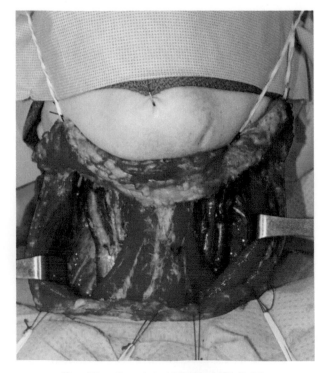

Fig. 15 Completed bilateral ND (I–V).

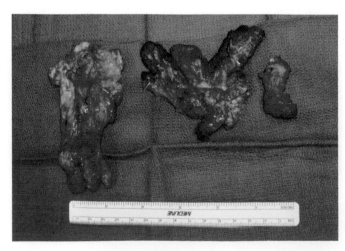

Fig. 17 Total thyroidectomy.

References

1. Gharib H, Goellner JR. Fine-needle aspiration biopsy of the thyroid: an appraisal. Ann Intern Med 1993;118:282—9.

2. Avenia N, Sanguinetti A, Cirocchi R, et al. Antibiotic prophylaxis in thyroid surgery: a preliminary multicentric Italian experience. Ann Surg Innov Res 2009;3:10.

3. Kern KA. Medicolegal analysis of errors in diagnosis and treatment of surgical endocrine disease. Surgery 1993;114:1167.

4. Hermann M, Alk G, Roka R, et al. Laryngeal recurrent nerve injury in surgery for benign thyroid diseases: effect of nerve dissection and impact of individual surgeon in more than 27,000 nerves at risk. Ann Surg 2002;235:261.

5. Randolph GW, Dralle H, International Intraoperative Monitoring Study Group, et al. Electrophysiologic recurrent laryngeal nerve monitoring during thyroid and parathyroid surgery: international standards guideline statement. Laryngoscope 2011; 121(Suppl 1):S1.

6. Randolph GW. Surgery of the thyroid and parathyroid glands. 2nd edition. Philadelphia: Saunders Elsevier; 2013.

7. Bononi M, Amore Bonapasta S, Vari A, et al. Incidence and circumstances of cervical hematoma complicating thyroidectomy and its relationship to postoperative vomiting. Head Neck 2010;32:1173.

8. Bellantone R, Lombardi CP, Raffaelli M, et al. Is routine supplementation therapy (calcium and vitamin D) useful after total thyroidectomy? Surgery 2002;132:1109.

Diagnosis and Management of Salivary Lesions of the Neck

Eric R. Carlson, DMD, MD

KEYWORDS

- Plunging ranula • Parotid tail tumor • Submandibular gland tumor • Submandibular gland mucocele • Submandibular sialolithiasis

KEY POINTS

- Salivary lesions of the neck comprise a variety of neoplastic and nonneoplastic processes. The determination of the involved gland and the exact pathologic process depends on a physical examination and a review of computed tomography (CT) scans or magnetic resonance imaging (MRI) of the neck.
- Once the salivary gland of origin of the neck mass is determined by physical examination and imaging review, the surgeon should determine whether fine-needle aspiration biopsy is required in preparation for removal of the pathologic entity.
- Benign parotid tail tumors are surgically managed by partial parotidectomy including facial nerve dissection and preservation; benign inferiorly located parotid tail tumors can occasionally be managed by extracapsular dissection without facial nerve identification.
- Malignant parotid tail tumors are typically managed with partial parotidectomy; malignant submandibular gland tumors are commonly managed with at least a 3-level prophylactic neck dissection that sacrifices the submandibular gland and tumor within the neck dissection.
- Fluid-filled lesions of the submandibular triangle are most commonly diagnosed as plunging ranulas and are typically managed by transoral excision of the etiologic sublingual gland; close scrutiny of the CT or MRI scans may reveal the presence of a submandibular gland mucocele that is managed by excision of the etiologic submandibular gland with or without associated sublingual gland excision.
- Chronic sialadenitis or sialolithiasis of the submandibular gland requires an assessment of the chronicity of the sialadenitis, the location of the sialoliths, and the likelihood of recovery of submandibular gland function when considering isolated excision of the submandibular sialoliths without excision of the submandibular gland.

Introduction

The diagnosis and management of masses of the neck require strict attention to obtaining a history and performing a physical examination so as to establish a differential diagnosis for the mass under consideration. The development of a differential diagnosis of a neck mass frequently includes neoplastic and nonneoplastic salivary lesions that are considered as a function of the age of the patient, the patient's history, and the clinician's physical examination of the patient. This exercise is particularly important because the surgeon must consider the role of fine-needle aspiration biopsy and imaging studies of the neck before providing definitive surgical therapy for the mass. The anatomic region of the mass of the neck also permits the surgeon to include or discard certain diagnoses. For example, most salivary lesions of the neck occur in the lateral upper neck region, and specifically in level IB (submandibular gland) and level IIA (parotid tail). While placing salivary lesions on the differential diagnosis of a neck mass, it is important to understand that incisional biopsies of such neck masses have no role to play in their management. It is therefore essential that surgeons rely on available preoperative measures, including the development of a comprehensive and orderly differential diagnosis, obtaining structural imaging studies, and performing a fine-needle aspiration biopsy as indicated so as to execute the proper surgical treatment plan. This article reviews salient features and the surgical management of the most commonly encountered salivary lesions of the neck, including the plunging ranula and submandibular gland mucocele, the parotid tail tumor, the submandibular gland tumor, and sialadenitis/sialolithiasis of the submandibular gland.

Plunging ranula and submandibular gland mucocele

Most ranulas of the floor of mouth are large extravasation mucoceles that arise from the sublingual gland and are lined by granulation tissue rather than epithelium. The ranula was first described in the sixteenth century and its curative surgical treatment was subsequently discussed in the seventeenth century. The exact tissue of origin of the ranula was elucidated in the nineteenth century, and its pathophysiologic mechanism was first clearly described in 1956. A lengthy treatise on the

Department of Oral and Maxillofacial Surgery, University of Tennessee Medical Center, The University of Tennessee Cancer Institute, 1930 Alcoa Highway, Suite 335, Knoxville, TN 37920, USA

E-mail address: ecarlson@mc.utmck.edu

Atlas Oral Maxillofacial Surg Clin N Am 23 (2015) 49-61
1061-3315/15/$ - see front matter © 2015 Elsevier Inc. All rights reserved.
http://dx.doi.org/10.1016/j.cxom.2014.10.005

surgical management of the ranula with sublingual gland excision was published in 1969. Clinical observation shows that some ranulas may descend into the submandibular triangle through a posteriorly located mylohyoid hiatus, or a herniation in the mylohyoid muscle, and are therefore referred to as plunging ranulas. Such plunging ranulas develop discrete neck masses that are appreciated on physical examination. Some investigators have indicated that repeated aspirations or conservative drainage procedures of oral ranulas encourage the development of scar tissue in the mucosa of the floor of mouth such that a plunging ranula develops in the neck as the path of least resistance. The anatomy of the mylohyoid muscle and its hiatus or cleft, and herniations within the mylohyoid muscle, have been studied to explain the development of plunging ranulas. In their study of 23 adult cadavers, Harrison and colleagues identified that a bilateral mylohyoid hiatus existed in 10 of their 23 specimens (43%), with the hiatus being unilateral in 6 (26%) and bilateral in 4 (17%) cadavers. The median anteroposterior dimension of the hiatus was 7 mm, with a range of 2 to 11 mm, and the median mediolateral dimension was 14 mm with a range of 7 to 20 mm. The investigators identified sublingual gland tissue in 9 hernias and fat in 6 hernias.

Although the diagnosis of the conventional, nonplunging ranula remains straightforward, its management has historically been variable and controversial, ranging from incision and marsupialization to sublingual gland excision. Most mucoceles are located in the lower lip and are treated with an excision of the mucocele and associated causal minor salivary gland tissue of the lower lip. Although the ranula of the floor of mouth is

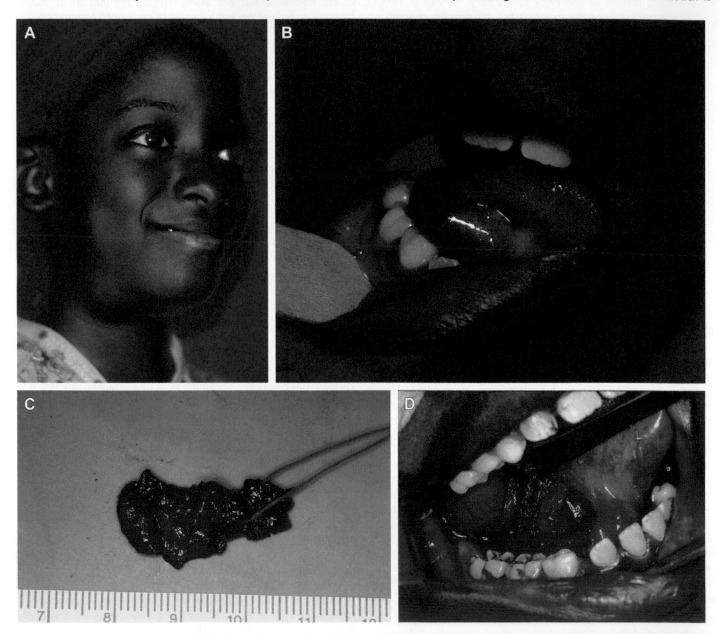

Fig. 1 A 9-year-old patient with a mass of the right neck (A) and an obvious ranula of the right floor of mouth (B). A clinical diagnosis of plunging ranula was therefore established. The patient was treated with sublingual gland excision (C) with identification and preservation of the right Wharton duct and lingual nerve in the floor of mouth (D) and without excision of the pseudocyst in the neck. The intraoperative forced expression of the saliva through the floor of mouth wound following sublingual gland removal permits postoperative resolution of the nonepithelial granulation tissue—lined pseudocyst. ([A, B] From Carlson ER, Ord RA. Cysts of the salivary glands. In: Carlson ER, Ord RA, editors. Textbook and color atlas of salivary gland pathology: diagnosis and management. Ames, Iowa: Wiley Blackwell; 2008; with permission.)

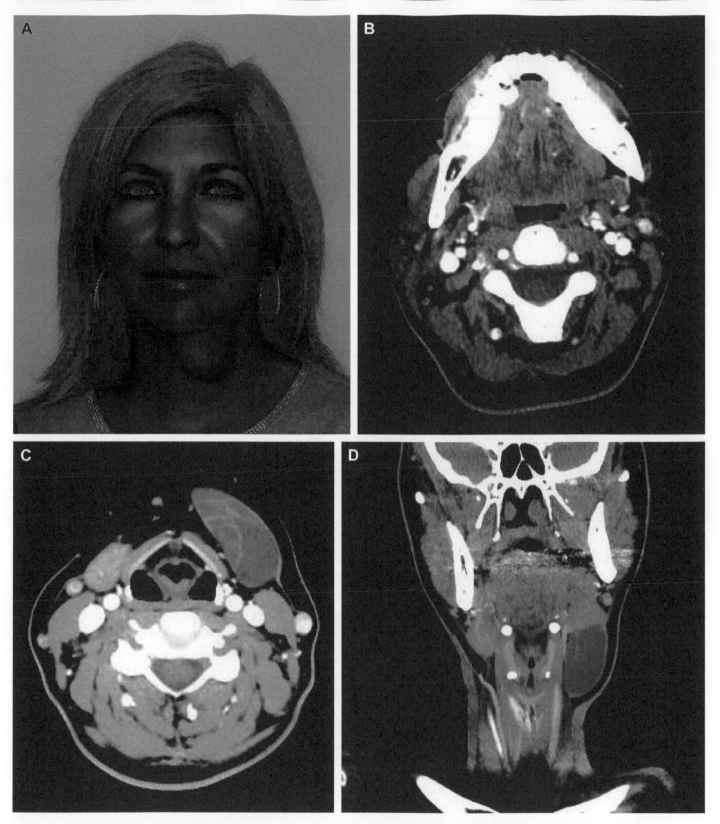

Fig. 2 A 37-year-old woman with a mass of level I of the left paramidline neck (*A*). Physical examination suggested a fluid-filled mass that supported a diagnosis of plunging ranula, although oral examination did not show findings consistent with this diagnosis. CT showed no tail sign of the sublingual gland region (*B*) although a fluid-filled mass was present in level I of the neck (*C*) that was intimately associated with the inferior aspect of the left submandibular gland (*D*). A provisional diagnosis of submandibular gland mucocele was therefore established. The patient underwent surgery with a transcutaneous approach to the left submandibular gland (*E*). The mucocele was dissected in the neck (*F*) and excised along with the left submandibular gland and left sublingual gland (*G*). Final pathology confirmed the diagnosis of submandibular gland mucocele (*H*; hematoxylin-eosin, original magnification × 200). The resultant defect is noted in the neck (*I*).

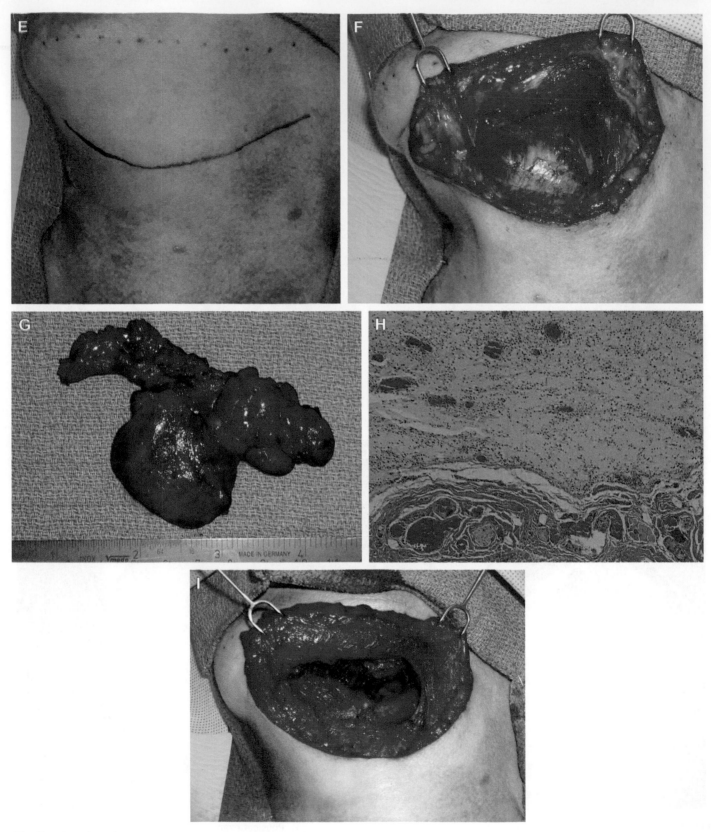

Fig. 2 (continued)

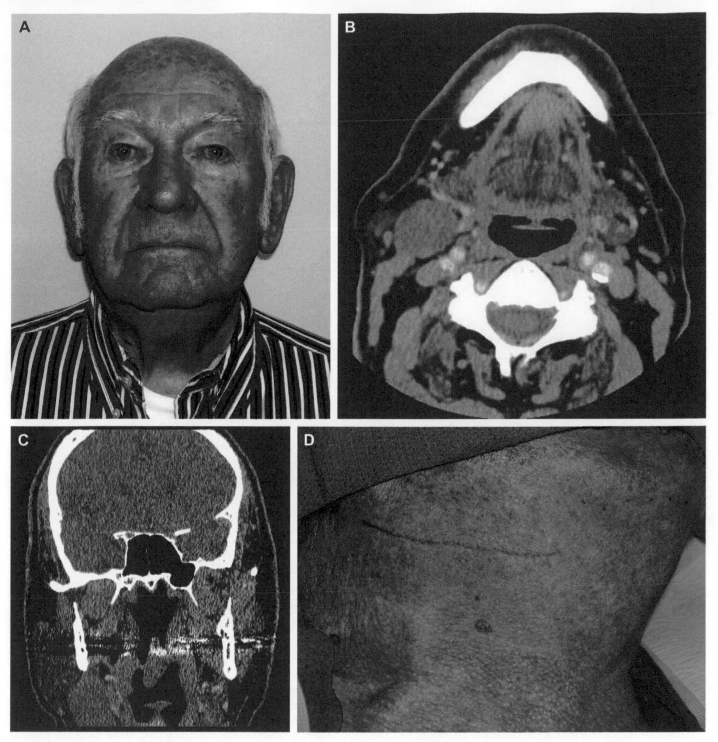

Fig. 3 An 83-year-old man with a mass of level II of the right neck (*A*). Physical examination revealed a discrete mass that was indurated but equivocal as to its tissue of origin. CT scans identified a homogeneous mass (*B*) that was associated with the tail of the right parotid gland (*C*). The patient underwent extracapsular dissection of the right parotid tail tumor through an upper neck incision (*D*) rather than a traditional modified Blair incision for parotid surgery. Careful extracapsular dissection was performed to identify the tumor's pseudo-capsule, thereby avoiding tumor spillage (*E*). The specimen is noted to consist of a pseudoencapsulated tumor with a portion of the tail of the right parotid gland at its superior surface (*F*). The bivalved specimen (*G*) shows signs consistent with pleomorphic adenoma, which is confirmed on histopathology (*H*; hematoxylin-eosin, original magnification × 4). The patient showed acceptable signs of healing, as noted 1 year after surgery (*I, J*).

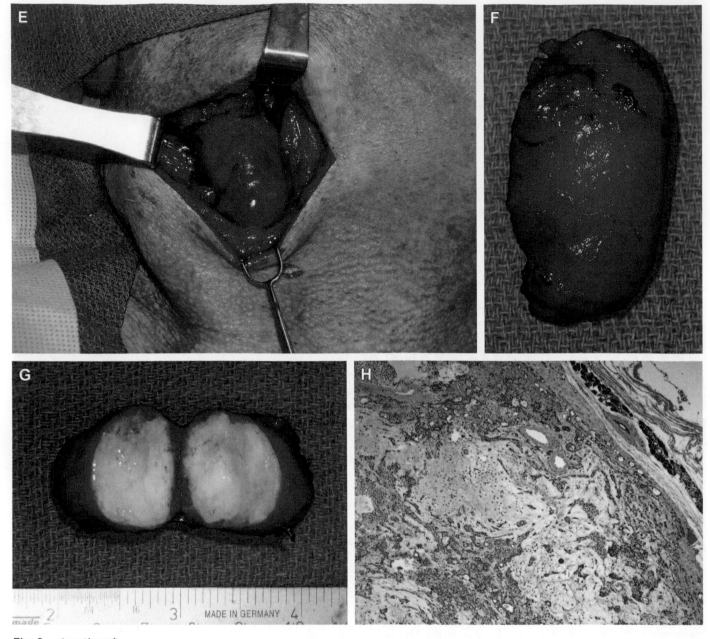

Fig. 3 *(continued)*

the second most common type of mucocele, removal of the ranula and the associated salivary gland (in this case, the sublingual gland) has not been uniformly accepted as standard treatment of the ranula as it is for the lower lip mucocele. The management of the plunging ranula has also been variably described, ranging from sclerotherapy to excision of the sublingual gland with or without ranula excision/submandibular gland excision. Excision of the etiologic sublingual gland with or without removal of the plunging ranula represents curative treatment in most cases (Fig. 1). A thorough knowledge of floor of mouth anatomy and its precise surgical dissection results in an uncomplicated surgical procedure and expedient cure of the plunging ranula. In terms of the specific dissection of the floor of mouth, the inferior surface of the sublingual gland is carefully separated from the underlying Wharton duct while the posterior-lateral surface of the gland is separated from the lingual nerve. The identification of these structures and their careful dissection is associated with little morbidity when

performing this surgical procedure. Any procedure less than excision of all or part of the sublingual gland is speculative in terms of a curative result of this diagnosis.

Clinical observation indicates that some patients present with a neck examination consistent with a diagnosis of plunging ranula, but without signs of ranula on oral examination. Moreover, many of these patients show CT evidence of the mucocele originating from the submandibular gland rather than from the sublingual gland. These rare cases are typically diagnosed as submandibular gland mucoceles and should be treated with excision of the etiologic submandibular gland and associated mucocele (Fig. 2). A thorough analysis of the CT scans is thought to be able to distinguish the sublingual gland ranula from the submandibular mucocele by identifying the tail-like extension of the ranula to the sublingual gland, which is absent in the submandibular gland mucocele. However, the management of the submandibular gland mucocele frequently involves removal of the submandibular gland and

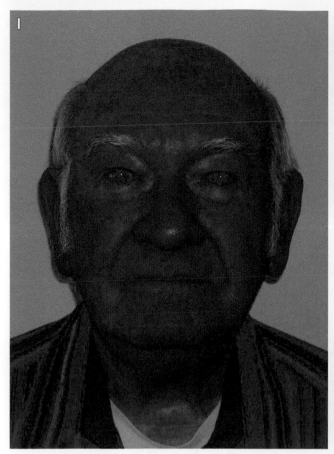
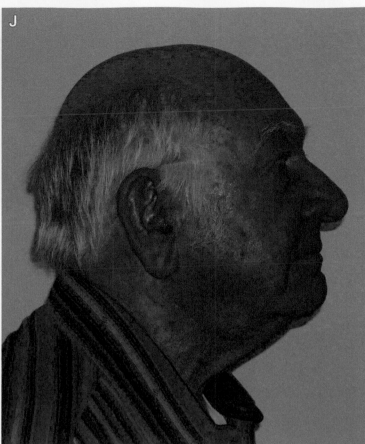

Fig. 3 (*continued*)

the sublingual gland and represents a curative procedure for this diagnosis. To this end, a transcutaneous dissection is accomplished and a subfascial approach to the submandibular gland excision is observed, with identification and ligation of the facial artery and vein. With inferior-posterior retraction of the submandibular gland, and with anterior retraction of the mylohyoid muscle, the lingual nerve is identified. The sublingual gland can be separated from the lingual nerve and both salivary glands are ultimately delivered. The mucocele is frequently able to be excised with the gland en bloc (see Fig. 2G).

Parotid tail tumor

For decades, superficial parotidectomy has represented the standard operation for removal of a tumor of the superficial lobe of the parotid gland, including those tumors derived from the parotid tail. During a superficial parotidectomy, the facial nerve is completely dissected and preserved and the entire parotid gland and tumor located superficial to the facial nerve are sacrificed. The surgeon may alternatively choose to perform a partial superficial parotidectomy whereby a cuff of normal parotid tissue is included at the periphery of the tumor and the facial nerve is dissected and preserved in the region of the gland's dissection and sacrifice. Regardless of whether a superficial parotidectomy or partial superficial parotidectomy is performed for benign tumors, a pseudocapsule on the deep surface of the tumor often separates the tumor from the facial nerve dissection. As such, marginal tumor resections and close

margins are expected in the area of the preserved facial nerve because an extracapsular dissection is performed in this area. Extensive study of the pseudocapsule adjacent to the facial nerve dissection has shown that the dissection of any thickness of pseudocapsule containing the tumor without intraoperative tumor spillage translates to a high likelihood of cure without recurrence. As such, salivary gland surgeons who preferentially perform the superficial parotidectomy or partial superficial parotidectomy frequently also incorporate an extracapsular dissection of parotid tumors while completing a thorough dissection and preservation of the facial nerve. It is therefore difficult to avoid the performance of at least a limited extracapsular dissection of most parotid tumors, particularly those tumors of the parotid tail.

The tail of the parotid gland is defined as the most inferior portion of the superficial lobe of the gland. It lies antero-lateral to the sternocleidomastoid muscle, posterolateral to the posterior belly of the digastric muscle, and inferior to the angle of the mandible. The parotid tail has been quantified as the inferior 2.0 cm of the gland. The management of the parotid tail tumor is an example of an extracapsular dissection being performed intentionally because the inferior extent of the parotid tail tumor extends beyond the confines of the parotid gland (Fig. 3). Some inferiorly located parotid tail tumors represent challenges for radiologists interpreting CT scans in an effort to diagnose the tissue of origin of a neck mass. It can be particularly difficult to diagnose parotid tail tumors based on axial scans alone such that coronal scans are required to determine the origin of the neck mass at the

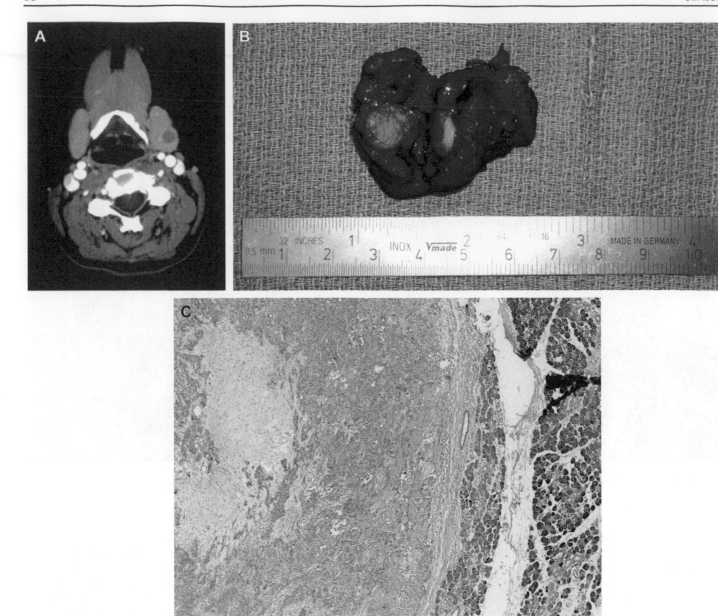

Fig. 4 CT scan of a pathologic process of the left submandibular gland (*A*). Preoperative fine-needle aspiration biopsy was performed and suggested benign neoplastic disease such that the patient was treated by submandibular gland excision (*B*). A pleomorphic adenoma was diagnosed (*C*; hematoxylin-eosin, original magnification × 4). CT scan showing a tumor of the right submandibular gland (*D*). A preoperative fine-needle aspiration biopsy identified malignancy within the submandibular gland such that the patient was treated with a selective neck dissection (I-III) that included the submandibular gland and tumor within the specimen (*E*). Final pathology documented undifferentiated adenoid cystic carcinoma in the submandibular gland with perineural and intraneural invasion (*F*; hematoxylin-eosin, original magnification × 10) and metastatic cancer in 4 of 32 cervical lymph nodes in the specimen.

parotid tail (see Fig. 3B, C). This determination is important before proceeding with excision of such a neck mass because without it the surgeon would otherwise proceed with an excision of the mass without the inclusion of the tail of the parotid gland. Such a maneuver predisposes patients to persistence of their tumors. The proper identification of the mass developing from the parotid tail therefore permits curative tumor surgery provided that tumor spillage does not occur during this extracapsular dissection. In terms of the specific type of parotid tail surgery, a low parotid tail tumor is unlikely to require identification of the facial nerve during a strictly extracapsular dissection of the parotid tail tumor with incorporation of a cuff of parotid tail. If a high parotid tail tumor is diagnosed, a partial parotidectomy with identification

of the main trunk of the facial nerve may be required. Under such circumstances, surgeons should proceed with the dissection using a nerve stimulator.

Submandibular gland tumor

Submandibular gland tumors are rare, accounting for only 10% of all salivary gland tumors, and only 2% of all head and neck tumors. In 1936, McFarland provided the first report of submandibular gland tumors with his treatise on 301 tumors of the major salivary glands, including 278 parotid tumors, 22 submandibular tumors, and 1 sublingual tumor. As in the author's 1933 publication, no specific comments regarding surgical technique were offered, including that for submandibular

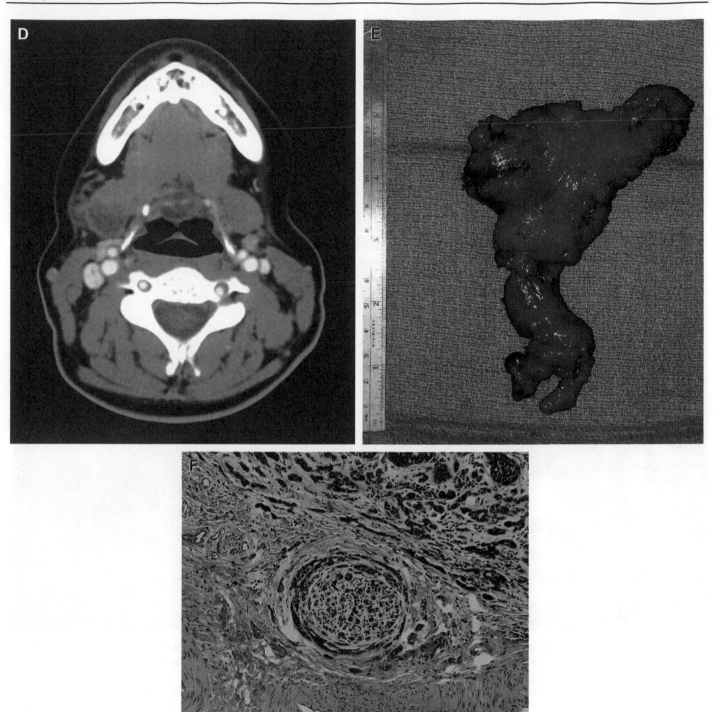

Fig. 4 (continued)

gland tumors, although the author indicated that 8 of the 22 submandibular gland tumors recurred. In 1953, Foote and Frazell first provided a specific assessment of the histologic diagnosis of 877 major salivary gland tumors, of which 107 were located in the submandibular gland. These submandibular gland tumors included 47 benign mixed tumors, 11 malignant mixed tumors, 17 adenoid cystic carcinomas, and 8 mucoepidermoid carcinomas, but specific mention was not made of the technical aspects of the surgery performed for removal of these tumors. It was not until 1966 that Work introduced comments regarding the surgical excision of major salivary glands associated with benign and malignant neoplastic diagnoses, and he was the first to recommend prophylactic neck dissection in the case of a primary submandibular gland malignancy.

When examining an enlarged submandibular gland, the more common nonneoplastic inflammatory and obstructive processes should initially be considered in the differential diagnosis. The international literature indicates that the ratio of nonneoplastic to neoplastic lesions of the submandibular gland is approximately 5:1. The presence of a discrete mass of the submandibular gland on physical examination typically suggests a neoplasm, whereas a diffuse swelling of the submandibular gland typically connotes an inflammatory process. In addition, when a neoplastic entity is diagnosed in the submandibular gland, the incidence of benign versus malignant

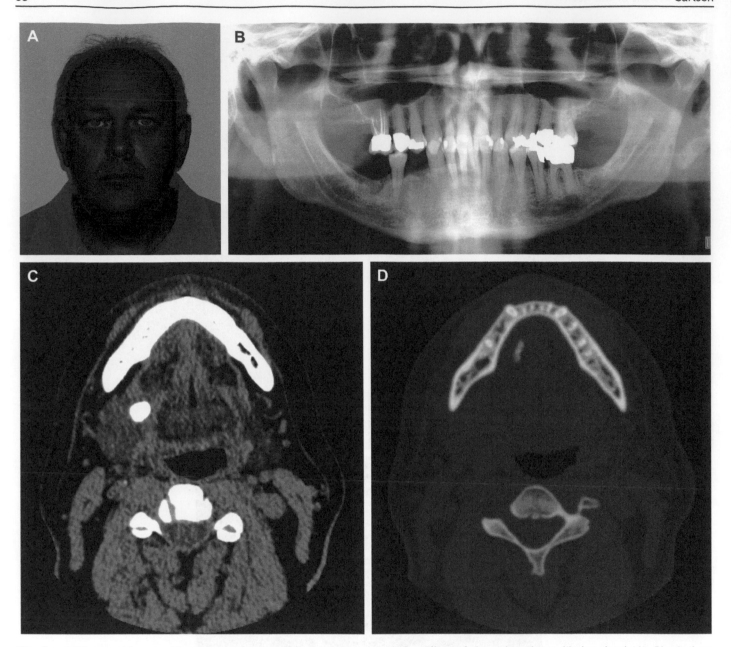

Fig. 5 A 50-year-old man with a 10-year history of intermittent pain and swelling of the right submandibular gland (*A*). Physical examination showed an indurated left submandibular gland that was tender to palpation such that a clinical diagnosis of sialadenitis was established. A panoramic radiograph (*B*) and CT scan showed a single intraglandular sialolith (*C*), and several extraglandular sialoliths (*D*). The patient underwent right submandibular gland excision (*E*, *F*) that permitted identification of the intraglandular stone at the hilum of the gland. Excision of the submandibular gland requires identification of the lingual nerve and the Wharton duct (*E*) with preservation of the nerve and proximal ligation of the duct. This excision requires attention to the marginal mandibular branch of the facial nerve, the anatomic position of which is not excessively retracted during the dissection. The patient also required removal of the distal extraglandular sialoliths through a transoral approach (*G*, *H*). Six extraglandular stones were identified (*I*). The duct was inspected for residual sialoliths at the conclusion of their removal (*J*). The patient's postoperative course was uncomplicated and his neck incision (*K*) and oral incision (*L*) are well healed, as noted 1 year after surgery.

diagnoses is similar such that preoperative assessment with fine-needle aspiration biopsy is required to determine the proper surgery for the submandibular gland tumor. For example, a cytologically benign process in the submandibular gland is managed by submandibular gland/tumor excision (Fig. 4A–C), whereas a malignant diagnosis in the submandibular gland is managed by neck dissection within which the submandibular gland is sacrificed (see Fig. 4D–F). Whether performing the surgery for a benign or malignant process, the

surgeon must pay particular attention to the soft tissues surrounding the tumor located within the submandibular gland so as to avoid tumor spillage during the dissection. The investing fascia is included with the malignant submandibular gland tumor as a standard principle involved in neck dissections. However, the technical aspects of a benign tumor excision are different. In such cases, a sufficient cuff of uninvolved investing fascia and/or tumor pseudocapsule should intentionally be included as an anatomic barrier on the specimen.

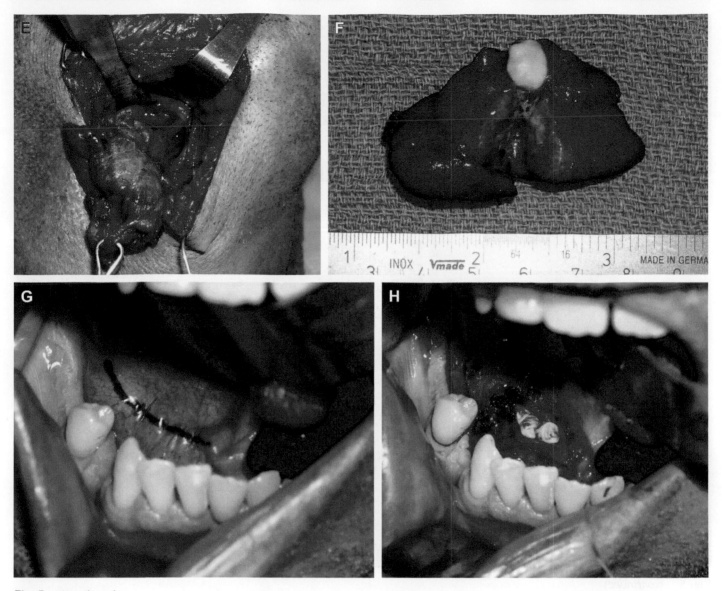

Fig. 5 (*continued*)

Submandibular sialadenitis/sialolithiasis

The evaluation of a patient with a diffuse, rather than discrete, swelling of the submandibular gland requires that the surgeon obtain a history regarding the chronicity of the swelling, whether the swelling increases during eating, whether the swelling is associated with pain, and the patient's medical comorbidity including the use of medications that might predispose the patient to sialadenitis. Whether because of scar tissue within the submandibular gland related to sialadenitis or because of the presence of a sialolith associated with the submandibular gland, the obstructive nature of either diagnosis results in a diffuse and commonly painful swelling of the submandibular gland. The physical examination of the patient should specifically assess for the presence of a discrete mass versus a diffuse swelling of the submandibular gland, the presence of tenderness to palpation of

These techniques of removal of benign and malignant submandibular gland tumors represent sound principles of tumor surgery.

the submandibular gland, the presence of cervical adenopathy, and the presence of pus at the distal end of the Wharton duct. While obtaining the patient's history and performing the physical examination of the neck, surgeons should keep in mind that sialadenitis is a more common, but not exclusive, diagnosis of a diffuse submandibular gland swelling compared with a benign or malignant tumor. In their assessment of 110 submandibular gland lesions, Gallia and Johnson determined that 15% of these swellings led to a diagnosis of neoplastic disease, whereas 85% were nonneoplastic, and 83% of the nonneoplastic lesions were ultimately diagnosed as sialadenitis. Overall, 91 of 110 submandibular gland swellings indicated sialadenitis. These statistics are in contrast with their 140 parotid gland lesions, of which 102 indicated neoplastic disease and 38 were caused by nonneoplastic disease, of which 24 were related to inflammatory disease.

When an empiric diagnosis of submandibular sialadenitis is established for a patient, the surgeon should obtain a panoramic radiograph to investigate for the presence of a sialolith. A screening panoramic radiograph is therefore indicated in all patients for whom a clinical diagnosis of sialadenitis of the submandibular gland has been established. When a

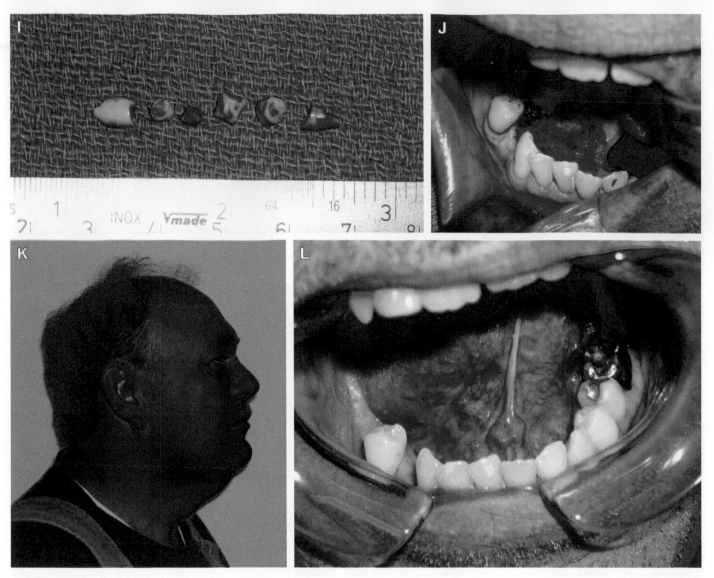

Fig. 5 (*continued*)

submandibular sialolith is noted on a panoramic radiograph, the surgeon is able to offer an expedient remedy to the patient's symptoms and diagnosis. However, 20% of submandibular sialoliths are radiolucent and therefore escape diagnosis with plain radiographs. In their review of 245 cases of sialolithiasis, Lustmann and colleagues found that 231 of these cases (94.3%) were present in the submandibular gland, 11 (4.5%) were present in the parotid gland, and 1 (0.4%) was present in the sublingual gland. Ninety-four percent of their 245 patients presented with swelling, 65.2% of their patients had pain, 15.5% had purulence, and 2.4% of their patients had no symptoms. Therefore, regardless of the patient's symptom complex, a clinical diagnosis of sialadenitis should result in the acquisition of a panoramic radiograph to determine whether a sialolith is responsible for the sialadenitis. If a sialolith is identified, the location of the stone dictates the appropriate surgical treatment (Fig. 5). The surgical approach to the submandibular gland excision for a diagnosis of sialadenitis or sialolithiasis is strictly subfascial with particular attention to effective ligation of the facial artery and vein, sacrifice of the submandibular ganglion while protecting the integrity of the lingual nerve, and proper protection of the anatomic location of the marginal mandibular branch of the facial nerve (see Fig. 5E).

Summary

Salivary lesions occupy a prominent position in the differential diagnosis of neck masses; particularly those located in level I and II of the neck. In most cases, the patient's history and physical examination and radiographic studies are able to strongly suggest the diagnosis. A fine-needle aspiration biopsy should be considered in the work-up of parotid tail masses and this biopsy should be obtained in the work-up of discrete masses of the submandibular gland noted on physical examination and confirmed by CT scans. This sequence of therapy results in precise and expedient surgical treatment of these neck masses.

Further readings

Anastassov GE, Haiavy J, Solodnick P, et al. Submandibular gland mucocele: diagnosis and management. Oral Surg Oral Med Oral Pathol Oral Radiol Endod 2000;89:159—63.

Bhaskar SN, Bolden TE, Weinmann JP. Pathogenesis of mucoceles. J Dent Res 1956;35:863—74.

Carlson ER, Ord RA, editors. Textbook and color atlas of salivary gland pathology — diagnosis and management. Ames (IA): Wiley-Blackwell Publishing; 2008.

Carlson ER, Webb D. The diagnosis and management of parotid pathology. Oral Maxillofac Surg Clin North Am 2013;25:31—48.

Carlson ER. Diagnosis and management of salivary gland infections. Oral Maxillofac Surg Clin North Am 2009;21:293—312.

Carlson ER. Differential diagnosis and management of neck masses. Chapter 25. In: Laskin DM, editor. Clinician's handbook of oral and maxillofacial surgery. Chicago: Quintessence Publishing Co; 2010. p. 370—8.

Catone GA, Merrill RG, Henny FA. Sublingual gland mucus-escape phenomenon — treatment by excision of sublingual gland. J Oral Surg 1969;27:774—86.

Dalgic A, Karakoc O, Karahatay S, et al. Submandibular triangle masses. J Craniofac Surg 2013;24:e529—30.

Foote FW, Frazell EL. Tumors of the major salivary glands. Cancer 1953; 4:1065—133.

Gallia LJ, Johnson JT. The incidence of neoplastic versus inflammatory disease in major salivary gland masses diagnosed by surgery. Laryngoscope 1981;91:512—6.

Gallina E, Gallo O, Boccuzzi S, et al. Analysis of 185 submandibular gland excisions. Acta Otorhinolaryngol Belg 1990;44:7—10.

Hamilton BE, Salzman KL, Wiggins RH, et al. Earring lesions of the parotid tail. AJNR Am J Neuroradiol 2003;24:1757—64.

Harrison JD, Kim A, Al-Ali S, et al. Postmortem investigation of mylohyoid hiatus and hernia: aetiological factors of plunging ranula. Clin Anat 2013;26:693—9.

Harrison JD. Modern management and pathophysiology of ranula: literature review. Head Neck 2010;32:1310—20.

Hze-Khoong EP, Xu L, Shen S, et al. Submandibular gland mucocele associated with a mixed ranula. Oral Surg Oral Med Oral Pathol Oral Radiol 2012;113:e6—9.

McFarland J. Three hundred mixed tumors of the salivary glands, of which sixty-nine recurred. Surg Gynecol Obstet 1936;63:457—68.

McGurk M, Eyeson J, Thomas B, et al. Conservative treatment of oral ranula by excision with minimal excision of the sublingual gland: histological support for a traumatic etiology. J Oral Maxillofac Surg 2008;66:2050—7.

Olubaniyi BO, Chow U, Mandalia S, et al. Evaluation of biopsy methods in the diagnosis of submandibular space pathology. Int J Oral Maxillofac Surg 2014;43:281—5. http://dx.doi.org/10.1016/j.ijom.2013.08.009.

Orabona GD, Bonavolonta P, Iaconetta G, et al. Surgical management of benign tumors of the parotid gland: extracapsular dissection versus superficial parotidectomy — our experience in 232 cases. J Oral Maxillofac Surg 2013;71:410—3.

Ozturk K, Yaman H, Arbag H, et al. Submandibular gland mucocele: report of two cases. Oral Surg Oral Med Oral Pathol Oral Radiol Endod 2005;100:732—5.

Patel MR, Deal AM, Shockley WW. Oral and plunging ranulas: what is the most effective treatment? Laryngoscope 2009;119:1501—9.

Rapidis AD, Stavrianos S, Lagogiannis G, et al. Tumors of the submandibular gland: clinicopathologic analysis of 23 patients. J Oral Maxillofac Surg 2004;62:1203—8.

Riffat F, Mahrous AK, Buchanan MA, et al. Safety of extracapsular dissection in benign superficial parotid lesions. J Maxillofac Oral Surg 2012;11:407—10.

Sigismund PE, Bozzato A, Schumann M, et al. Management of ranula: 9 years' clinical experience in pediatric and adult patients. J Oral Maxillofac Surg 2013;71:538—44.

Vaidhyanath R, Harieaswar S, Kendall C, et al. Pleomorphic adenoma arising from the tail of the parotid gland — value of preoperative multi planar imaging: a case report. Cases J 2008;1:1.

Venkat Suresh B, Vora SK. Huge plunging ranula. J Maxillofac Oral Surg 2012;11:487—90.

Work WP. Therapy of salivary gland tumors. Arch Otolaryngol 1966; 83:31—3.

Vascular Anomalies of the Neck

David E. Webb, Maj, USAF, DC [a],*, Joseph McDermott, MD [b],
David Grover, MD [c]

KEYWORDS

- Vascular anomalies • Head and neck surgery • Embolization • Imaging

KEY POINTS

- The key to good surgery is good access, and the key to good access is good surgery. This is never more true than when dealing with vascular lesions—which demand unrestricted exposure.
- Hypervascular tumors or those known to have a high degree of blood loss during surgery may benefit from preoperative embolization.
- If embolization is necessary, the embolic agent can be determined by using the following 3-question algorithm:
  - Is the vessel to be embolized large or small?
  - How long (temporally) is the vessel to remain occluded?
  - Is the tissue supplied by the vessel to remain viable after the embolization?
- Surgery is usually performed the day after embolization, although some investigators suggest resection can be delayed up to 8 days.

 Video of the flammable nature of Onyx during electrocautery of the post-embolized facial artery accompanies this article at http://www.oralmaxsurgeryatlas.theclinics.com/

Introduction

A multidisciplinary team is imperative to the diagnosis and successful management of vascular anomalies of the head and neck. Patients routinely require the services of a radiologist (both imager and proceduralist) and an experienced surgeon. Hematologist-oncologists and dermatologists can also be of assistance. A patient's history cannot be overemphasized, as it aids the radiologist in deciding on imaging modalities, tailoring studies to the needs of the patient, and making the diagnosis.

This article discusses the classification of vascular anomalies, provides a clinicopathologic review of a few vascular lesions, reviews imaging principles of vascular anomalies and image-guided (interventional) procedures, and concludes with treatment pearls.

Classification of vascular anomalies

The whole team should share a common lexicon. The International Society for the Study of Vascular Anomalies (ISSVA)

provides such a framework for classifying "Vascular Tumors." These tumors, along with common examples, are listed in Table 1.

In addition to these vascular lesions, this article also considers "vascular-like tumors": hypervascular neoplasia such as hemangiopericytomas, paragangliomas (carotid body tumors and glomus tumors), and hypervascular metastasis.

Clinicohistopathologic description

Hemangiomas

Hemangiomas are common, comprising 7% of benign pediatric age tumors and affecting 4.5% of children. One-third of hemangiomas are found in the head and neck, and 14% within the oral cavity. Hemangiomas of childhood are divided into infantile and congenital types, based on whether they are fully developed at birth. Hemangiomas that develop in adulthood tend to be small and are often located within the oral cavity or pharynx. Mucosal hemangiomas develop in areas that are often traumatized, such as the lip, buccal mucosa, and tongue (Figs. 1–5).

Infantile hemangiomas

Infantile hemangiomas are the most common vascular neoplasms, and include capillary and cavernous hemangiomas of any organs. These hemangiomas develop more often in infants who are female, Caucasian, premature, or of low birth weight. Most infantile hemangiomas present between 2 weeks and 2 months after delivery, and grow with the child; they present as an erythematous macule, patch, or plaque, but may also be present within deep soft tissues. Most do not require medical

The views expressed in this material are those of the authors, and do not reflect the official policy or position of the US Government, the Department of Defense, or the Department of the Air Force.

[a] Department of Oral and Maxillofacial Surgery, David Grant USAF Medical Center, 101 Bodin Circle/SGDD, Travis AFB, CA 94535, USA
[b] Department of Pathology, David Grant USAF Medical Center, 101 Bodin Circle/SGQC, Travis AFB, CA 94535, USA
[c] Department of Radiology, David Grant USAF Medical Center, 101 Bodin Circle/SGQX, Travis AFB, CA 94535, USA
* Corresponding author.
E-mail address: david.webb.5@us.af.mil

Table 1 ISSVA classification for vascular anomalies

	Vascular Tumors		Vascular Malformations	
Benign	Locally Aggressive or Borderline	Malignant	Simple	Combined
Infantile hemangioma	Kaposiform hemangioendothelioma	Angiosarcoma	CM	CVM
Congenital hemangioma	Retiform hemangioendothelioma	Epithelioid	LM	CLM
Rapidly involuting (RICH)	Papillary intralymphatic angioendothelioma	hemangioendothelioma	VM	CAMV
Noninvoluting (NICH)	(PILA), Dabska tumor		AVM	LVM
Partially involuting (PICH)	Composite hemangioendothelioma		AVF	CLVM
Tufted angioma	Kaposi sarcoma			CLAVM
Spindle-cell hemangioma				CVAVM
Epithelioid hemangioma				CLVAVM
Pyogenic granuloma (lobular capillary hemangioma)				

Abbreviations: AV, arteriovenous; C, capillary; F, fistula; L, lymphatic; M, malformation; V, venous.

or surgical intervention. For those requiring medical intervention, propranolol and glucocorticoids are often the first-line therapy.

Capillary hemangiomas are the most common soft-tissue neoplasm in infants and children, and consist of numerous intertwining capillary-sized blood vessels. These tumors grow rapidly in first year of life, then undergo gradual involution over the next 1 to 7 years. By age 7, 75% to 90% regress.

Cavernous hemangiomas are composed of larger vascular spaces filled with erythrocytes, are generally larger than capillary hemangiomas, and may involve deeper tissue. Although they are usually well circumscribed, they may be locally destructive. Unlike capillary-type infantile hemangiomas, they do not spontaneously regress.

Congenital hemangiomas
Congenital hemangiomas are much rarer than infantile hemangiomas. Unlike infantile hemangiomas they are fully formed at birth, occur equally in males and females, and stain negative for GLUT1 by immunohistochemistry. Congenital hemangiomas occur as solitary lesions on the head or near limb joints, and are categorized by the tendency to spontaneously involute. Rapidly involuting congenital hemangiomas regress completely within 2 years of birth; noninvoluting congenital hemangiomas grow proportionately with the infant and may display partial involution, but not full regression.

Vascular malformations

Vascular malformations are vascular proliferations arising from disordered angiogenesis, either during development or following trauma, and are categorized as either high-flow lesions, which involve an artery, or low-flow lesions, which do not. Vascular malformations may also be categorized by the number of vessel types involved (see Table 1). Simple malformations are composed of only a single type of vessel, and

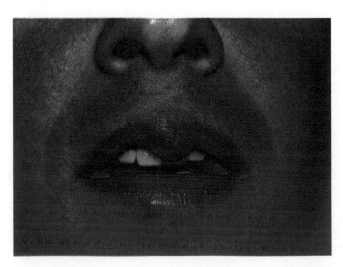

Fig. 1 A 40-year-old man presents with remote history of lip trauma. The lesion is firm and nonpulsatile.

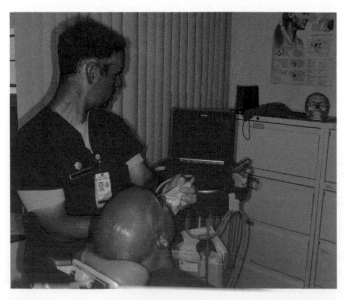

Fig. 2 In-office ultrasonography (US) performed to rule out a high-flow lesion/arterialization before incisional biopsy.

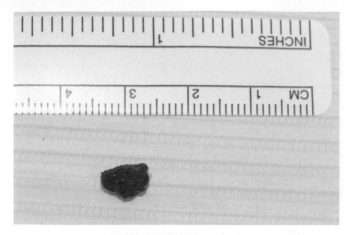

Fig. 3 Incisional biopsy yielded a diagnosis of hemangioma.

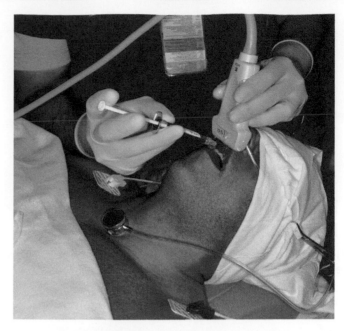

Fig. 5 Ultrasound-guided percutaneous sclerotherapy using 1.25% ethanolamine oleate during intravenous sedation.

combined malformations include any combination of capillary, lymphatic channel, artery, and vein.

High-flow lesions include arteriovenous fistulas (AVFs) and arteriovenous malformations (AVMs). AVFs develop following trauma, and consist of 1 or more shunts between arteries and other vascular structures. AVMs of the head and neck are serious lesions of unclear pathogenesis that are difficult to diagnose, treat, and cure; they may represent a spectrum of diseases rather than a single disease process. Most are present at time of birth, although they may present clinically several years later. Destructive lesions that grow throughout life and may have sudden, dramatic increases in size, AVMs may present clinically as a blush, similar to an early port-wine stain, which may have a pulse and thickening of the tissue, but no fluctuance.

In contrast to AVMs and AVFs, venous malformations (Figs. 6–10) are low-flow vascular malformations consisting of dilated veins. Venous malformations are rare, affecting 1 in 10,000 people, and often occur in the head and neck, involving the mucosa, skin, or muscle. Although most cases arise sporadically, they may arise secondary to an autosomal dominant disorder linked to chromosome 9P, or as part of a syndrome. Clinically they may present with pain or swelling and, unlike lymphangiomas, are compressible.

Lymphatic malformations

Lymphatic malformations are congenital dilatations of the lymphatic channels that may be categorized as microcystic,

macrocystic, or combined. Macrocystic lesions have a better prognosis, and are easier to treat, than microcystic lesions. The lesions may be focal, multifocal, or diffuse; they typically grow slowly, but may enlarge rapidly during puberty or at times of infection. Three-fourths of lymphatic malformations occur in the head and neck (Fig. 11).

Macrocystic lymphatic malformations (formerly known as cavernous lymphangiomas or cystic hygromas) may arise anywhere, but most often present as a painless, translucent soft mass underlying normal skin, within the posterior and anterior triangles of the lateral neck. Two-thirds of cases are recognized at the time of birth. These lesions may be associated with chromosomal abnormalities, such as Turner

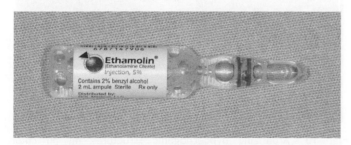

Fig. 4 Ethanolamine oleate is an example of a liquid sclerosing agent. (QOL Medical, LLC, Vero Beach, FL, USA.)

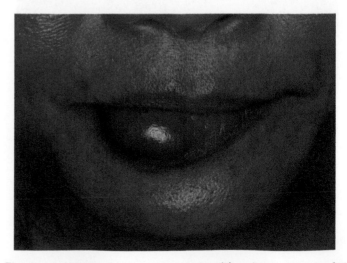

Fig. 6 A 41-year-old woman presents with a 4-year history of a spontaneous, gradually expanding lower lip mass. The patient complained of pain (7/10) and noted periodic fluctuations in size and color (ranging from *pink* to *purple*).

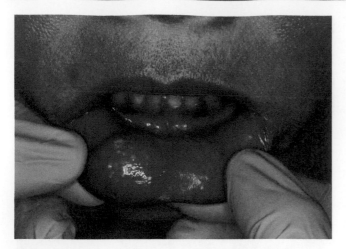

Fig. 7 Physical examination revealed a 2-cm diffuse mass, mildly tender to palpation, unaccompanied with a bruit or thrill.

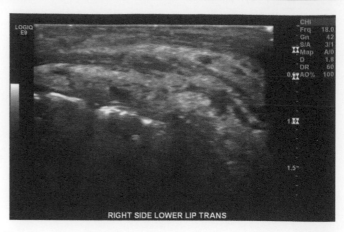

Fig. 9 US examination of the lower lip revealed a generally hyperechogenic mass with intermixed hypoechogenic arborizing structures.

syndrome and Down syndrome, or with other anomalies such as thyroglossal duct cyst. Complications include infection, hemorrhage, or compression of adjacent structures, causing difficulties with swallowing or speech. Because they may undergo spontaneous involution in infancy, surgery for infantile cases without complication should be postponed until age 3 to 5 years.

Hemangioendothelioma

Hemangioendotheliomas (HEs) are a group of rare proliferative vascular neoplasms, with behavior and histologic appearance intermediate between benign hemangiomas and malignant angiosarcoma. Of the several subtypes that exist, the most aggressive variety is epithelioid HE. Epithelioid HEs most often

arise as a poorly circumscribed mass near medium-sized vessels in young adults, expanding outwardly from the vessels, and obliterating the lumen. Old lesions may ossify and thus can be seen radiographically. Because they are rare tumors, without distinctive clinical or radiographic features, the diagnosis is usually unsuspected until histologic examination. Although they are generally indolent, almost one-third of epithelioid HEs metastasize to regional lymph nodes, lung, or bone, and 15% of patients die of the disease.

Kaposi sarcoma

Kaposi sarcoma (KS) is a rare malignancy of endothelial cells. Four types have been described: classic KS (found in Mediterranean men, involving the skin of the head and neck in 85% of cases, and rarely involving mucosa); human immunodeficiency virus—related KS (a widely invasive sarcoma involving skin in most cases, and involving the upper airway mucosa in nearly

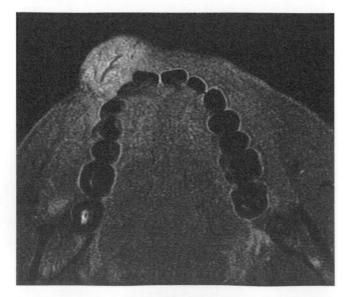

Fig. 8 Axial T2-weighted MRI shows a hyperintense venous malformation with prominent vascular channels. High-resolution T2-weighted sequences allow differentiation between low-flow and high-flow lesions.

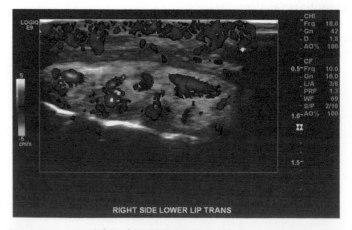

Fig. 10 Arborizing hypoechogenic structures fill on color Doppler, confirming vascular flow. Waveforms (not shown) were venous in nature, consistent with a venous malformation.

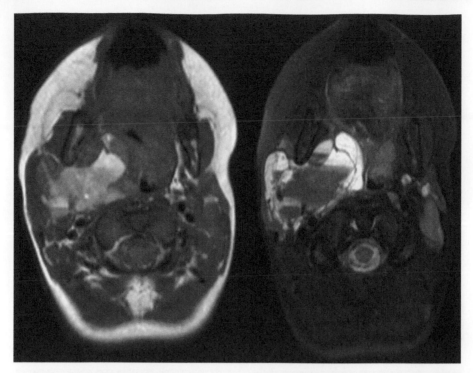

Fig. 11 (*Left*) Axial T1-weighted MRI with mixed-intensity mass in the right parapharyngeal space. (*Right*) Axial T2-weighted MRI with similar mixed-intensity mass, better delineating fluid-fluid levels, and septation. This low-flow vascular malformation is consistent with a lymphatic malformation.

one-fifth of cases); endemic KS (seen in sub-Saharan Africa); and iatrogenic KS (found in immunosuppressed organ transplant patients).

Skin lesions range from a solitary pale, erythematous macule, papule, or plaque, to widely disseminated purple-brown nodules. In the oral cavity, early-stage KS presents as erythematous, bluish, or dark brown macules, whereas later-stage disease appears as nodular or ulcerating lesions. Because of high recurrence rates, complete cure may be an unrealistic expectation for many patients. Solitary lesions may be treated by surgical excision, whereas extensive, multifocal lesions demand treatment with radiation and chemotherapy.

Angiosarcoma

Angiosarcoma is a diffusely infiltrative malignant vascular neoplasm with a dismal prognosis. It is the third most common head and neck sarcoma (following malignant fibrous histiocytoma and KS), accounting for 10% of head and neck sarcomas. Although they are extremely rare, comprising less than 1% of all sarcomas, more than half of all angiosarcomas are in the head and neck. Nearly three-quarters of head and neck angiosarcomas involve the skin, subcutaneous tissue, or deep tissue, with the remaining quarter involving the upper aerodigestive tract. Risk factors include history of radiation exposure, trauma, and chronic lymphedema. Most cases arise in patients with no risk factors. Angiosarcomas of the skin or mucosa present clinically as solitary or multifocal, red to blue hemorrhagic nodules. The clinical appearance may be indistinguishable from that of a pyogenic granuloma.

Hemangiopericytoma

Hemangiopericytoma (HPC) is an entity with considerable controversy regarding whether it exists as a distinct entity. The recent trend has been to reclassify tumors previously diagnosed as HPCs as solitary fibrous tumors. HPCs are rare, highly vascular soft-tissue tumors, with spindled to oval cells arranged around prominent, thin-walled blood vessels; they are found in all age groups but occur most often in middle-aged and older adults (Figs. 12–25). Although they may occur at any site, the head and neck is uncommon. Most head and neck HPCs develop in the upper aerodigestive tract, and 28% develop in the neck. Clinically, within the oral cavity HPCs typically present as a soft, rubbery, painless, rapidly enlarging, and well-demarcated red or bluish mass. Most HPCs are clinically benign. A meta-analysis of 116 cases of head and neck HPCs found that following surgery 28% recurred, and 6% recurred more than once. Overall rate of metastasis was 15%, with an average delay of 45 months from treatment of the primary lesion. Seventy-five percent of HPCs in the head and neck had a good prognosis following surgery, and overall 10-year survival rate was 90%. Adverse prognostic indicators include size greater than 5.0 cm, nonsurgical treatment, deep location, and poor histologic differentiation.

Paraganglioma

Paraganglioma (PG) is a rare, highly vascular neuroendocrine tumor, arising from parasympathetic ganglia such as the carotid body or vagus paraganglia, and usually associated with the great vessels of the head and neck (Figs. 26–32). PGs

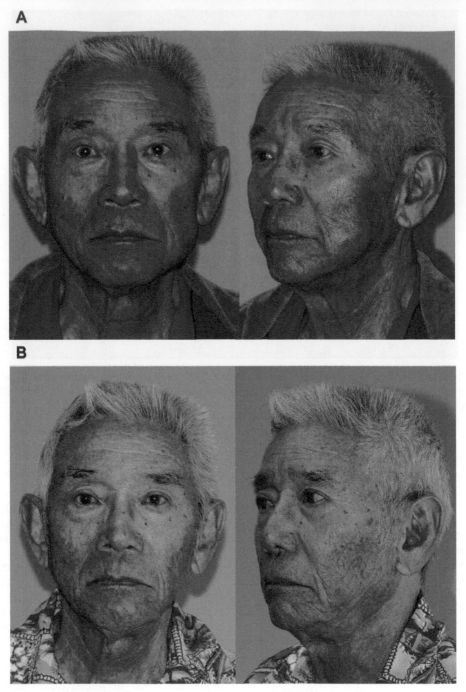

Fig. 12 (*A*) A 79-year-old man with a 4-month history of progressively enlarging left-sided facial swelling. The mass was rubbery, and without bruit or thrill. (*B*) One year post-operative result.

generally present in middle-aged adults (mean age 41–47 years). More than 30% of cases are hereditary, arising from hereditary paraganglioma syndrome, multiple endocrine neoplasia 2 syndrome, neurofibromatosis type 1, and Carney's triad. Most PGs are discovered through their mass effects on cranial nerves IX and X. PGs are found incidentally only 10% of the time. Less than 10% release catecholamines detected through biochemical blood testing. One study showed that over a period of 5 years, one-fifth of PGs decreased in size while the remainder either grew slowly (38%) or remained stable (42%). Surgery is the favored method of treatment when possible, and complete excision is possible in 90% to 97% of cases.

Imaging principles of vascular anomalies

The reader is referred to an article elsewhere in this issue by Brennan and Tilley for a more comprehensive discussion of the radiology of all neck masses. This section focuses only on the imaging of vascular lesions, with a general overview of each modality.

Plain (conventional) radiography

Plain, or conventional, radiography is useful when evaluating for the presence of phleboliths, secondary hypertrophy, or

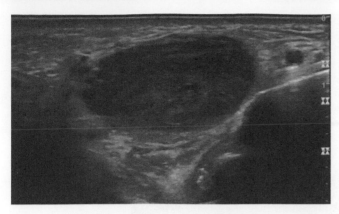

Fig. 13 In-office US showed a circumscribed, homogeneous, 3-cm soft-tissue mass. Elastography revealed a mixed density lesion.

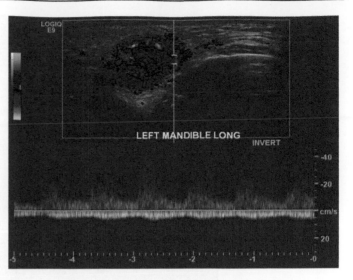

Fig. 15 Doppler waveform demonstrating arterialization of the mass. Fine-needle aspiration biopsy was inconclusive.

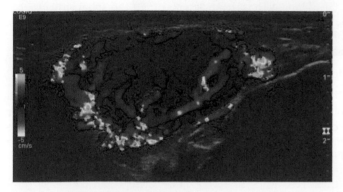

Fig. 14 Doppler US of the soft-tissue mass showing extensive vascularity to and of the lesion.

cortical changes of associated osseous structures, and as the initial study in evaluating for metastatic disease when applicable. Although inexpensive and easy to accomplish, plain radiography is insensitive, exposes the patient to ionizing radiation (especially concerning with pediatric patients), and is of limited utility.

Ultrasonography

Ultrasonography (US) plays a significant role in the evaluation of vascular anomalies. US allows for measurement of lesion size and depth, classification of the lesion as vascular, and differentiation

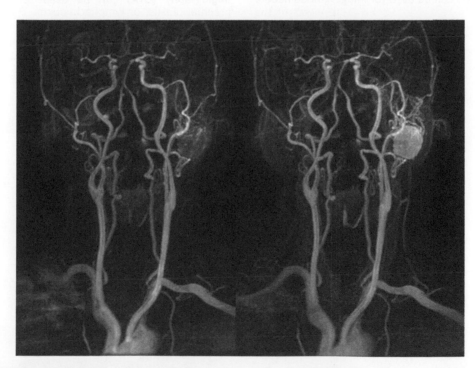

Fig. 16 Magnetic resonance angiography (MRA) of the head, neck, and upper thorax, showing early enhancement of the left juxta-mandibular vascular lesion.

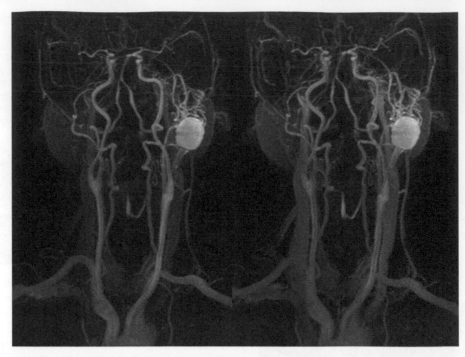

Fig. 17   MRA in later phase shows continued enhancement and early filling of the draining veins.

of cystic and solid components. Doppler interrogation is used to classify the vascular lesion as low-flow or high-flow (lesions are considered high-flow if an arterial component is present). Benefits of US include general availability (office or bedside), lack of ionizing radiation, and assessment of physiology. US issues include the need for an experienced sonographer, difficulty in differentiating tissue types, which makes size and depth measurements problematic, and the inability of sound waves to image through bone, metal, and air. Although US can demonstrate lesion proximity to vital structures, it is not the best modality for such. Lastly, US can be used for image-guided needle

placement for questionable lesions that require fine-needle or core biopsy, in addition to needle placement and procedure monitoring during percutaneous sclerotherapy injection (see Figs. 2, 5, 9, 10, 13–15).

Computed tomography and computed tomographic angiography

Computed tomography (CT) and computed tomographic angiography (CTA) can be used to measure lesion size,

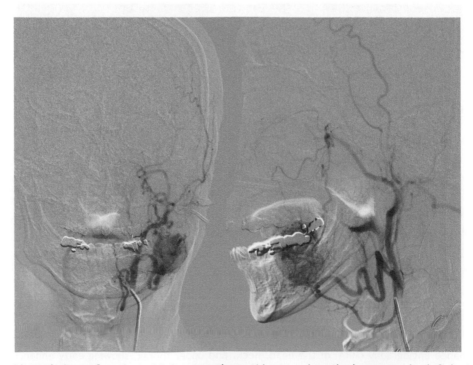

Fig. 18   Frontal and lateral views of a selected left external carotid artery show the hypervascular left juxtamandibular lesion.

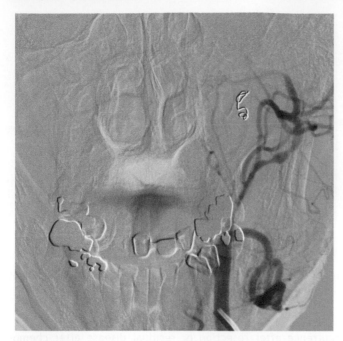

Fig. 19 Postembolization selected left external carotid angiogram shows lack of flow to lesion, and absence of enhancement. Lesional flow was accomplished with a combination of coil (left internal maxillary artery) and particulate (left facial artery) embolization.

determine invasiveness and secondary effects of the primary lesion, and assess for metastatic disease. In general, any question answered by plain radiography can be better answered by CT, at the cost of more ionizing radiation. The addition of iodinated contrast material improves lesion characterization and vessel evaluation. CTA can be used to determine which vessels are involved with a lesion and to help plan interventions. It is not the imaging modality of choice given its relative inability to differentiate soft tissues

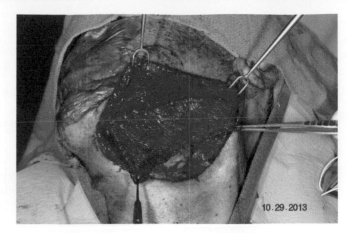

Fig. 21 Platysmal flap raised for postexcisional biopsy reconstruction.

(especially in infiltrative lesions) in comparison with MRI, but may be the only option in patients with contraindications to MRI (eg, pacemakers).

Magnetic resonance imaging

MRI is the study of choice for vascular lesions. Superior soft-tissue differentiation allows for the best characterization of the lesion as regards types of tissue, size, and depth, and effects on adjacent important structures (see Fig. 11 for a classic example of a low-flow vascular [lymphatic] malformation). Magnetic resonance angiography (MRA), either with or without gadolinium-based intravenous contrast, is able to evaluate adjacent vascular structures to determine physiology of the lesion, and can be used for procedural planning (see Figs. 16 and 17). Postprocedure issues, including evaluation of residual nidus after embolization and residual tumor after resection, are best accomplished by MRI (usually with contrast).

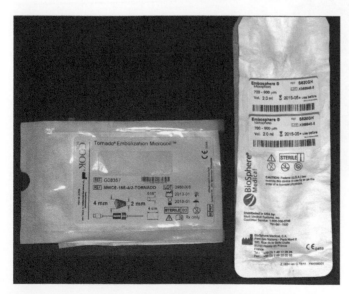

Fig. 20 Embolic materials used (coil and particle). (Cook, Inc., Bloomington, IN; and Merit Medical, S.A., Roissy-en-France, France).

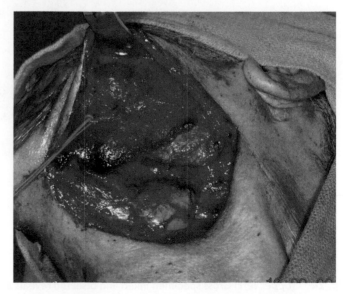

Fig. 22 Vessel loop identifying facial artery feeding into the mass.

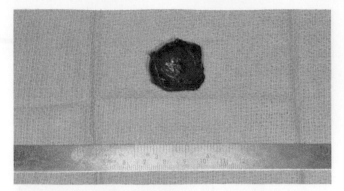

Fig. 23 Excisional biopsy of the encapsulated mass.

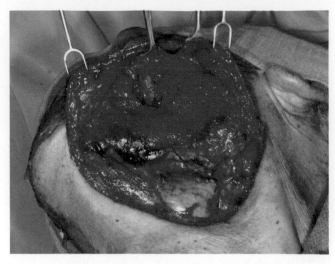

Fig. 25 Postexcisional biopsy defect reconstructed with a combination of buccal fat pad and superiorly based platysma flap.

Conventional angiography

Conventional angiography has a limited role, mostly as a troubleshooter when MRI/MRA is equivocal, or as part of an endovascular treatment. It is costly, invasive, and risks stroke when working in the head and neck. Detailed discussions with patients and angiographers should be undertaken when considering this modality.

Positron emission tomography combined with computed tomography

PET combined with CT has a limited role in the evaluation of vascular lesions. It is not generally used to evaluate the primary lesion but is the modality of choice when evaluating for metastatic disease. It also has an emerging role in post-therapy evaluation of malignant lesions (ie, detection of local

recurrence after resection or residual disease after chemotherapy or radiation therapy).

Image-guided (interventional) procedures

Image-guided procedures include fine-needle or core-needle biopsy, percutaneous sclerotherapy, and endovascular embolization. Needle biopsy is self-explanatory, with image guidance only sometimes necessary. This section reviews embolic materials, followed by an overview of image-guided procedures.

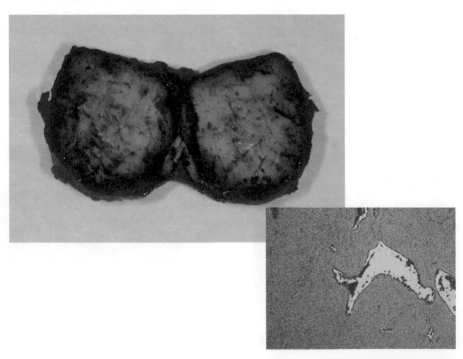

Fig. 24 (*Upper left*) Gross specimen inked and bisected reveals a fleshy-appearing surface with minute channels. (*Lower right*) Histology revealed a highly vascular neoplasm (note the classic staghorn-like vascular channel) consistent with solitary fibrous tumor/hemangiopericytoma. (Hematoxylin and Eosin, original magnification ×4)

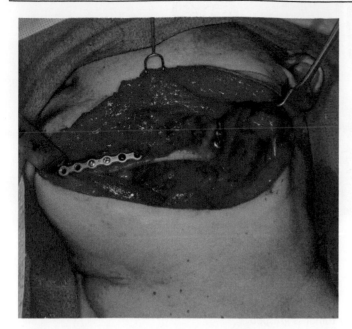

Fig. 26 Application of bone plates to index occlusion before performing an Attia double mandibular osteotomy to provide access for a paraganglioma (carotid body tumor).

Material overview

Particles

Particles used for permanent vessel occlusion occlude the vessel, which results in flow stasis and eventual thrombosis. The particles also incite an inflammatory response, enhancing the permanence of occlusion. Particles range in size from 100 to 1200 μm, and are produced in approximately 200-μm ranges (eg, 100–300 μm). Particles less than 300 μm in size are usually considered when embolizing small vessels. The smaller the particle, the more likely the embolization will lead to ischemia or even necrosis of the distal organ or tissue. Radiolucent particles are mixed with iodinated contrast and carefully injected via small syringes under fluoroscopic guidance. Particles can be made from polyvinyl alcohol or trisacryl gelatin.

Liquid adhesives

Liquid adhesives are agents that rapidly polymerize on exposure to ionic environments (eg, saline, blood), the most commonly used being cyanoacrylates (glues) such as n-butyl cyanoacrylate. Glues are mixed with ethiodized oil (radiopaque) before embolization; the mixture ratio influences the speed of polymerization. The level of embolization (usually small vessels) is determined by the speed of polymerization, catheter positioning, and blood flow. The glue creates an endoluminal cast of the targeted vascular bed leading to vessel blockage and inflammation, thus providing permanent vessel occlusion. Ethylene vinyl alcohol copolymer (also known as Onyx) is a foam-like adhesive used similarly to the cyanoacrylates, leading to intravascular cast formation and permanent vessel occlusion (Figs. 33, 34). The clinical significance of Onyx flammable nature is apparent in Video 1 available online at http://www.oralmaxsurgeryatlas.theclinics.com/).

Liquid sclerosants

Liquid sclerosants are agents that produce thrombosis and inflammation at the level of small vessels, leading to permanent vessel occlusion. The most robust agent is absolute ethanol, which leads to nearly instantaneous vessel thrombosis and cell death. Ethanol (radiolucent alone) can be mixed with contrast, but is no longer "absolute" and diminishes effectiveness. It can be delivered percutaneously via direct needle stick into lesions (see Figs. 4 and 5) or endovascularly via a catheter. Controlling the sclerosant flow within vascular lesions is imperative to effectively destroy the targeted lesion while minimizing nontarget embolization. Milder sclerosants include detergents (eg, sodium tetradecyl sulfate, polidocanol, sodium morrhuate, and ethanolamine oleate), osmotic agents such as hypertonic saline (23.4%), chemical irritants such as chromated glycerin (not approved by the Food and Drug Administration), and boiling contrast. The detergents, particularly sodium tetradecyl sulfate and polidocanol, are the agents of choice in the United States.

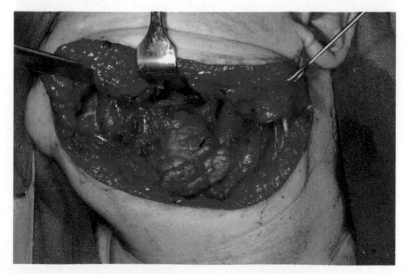

Fig. 27 Cephalad retraction of the osteotomized mandible provides access to the tumor. Note the preserved external jugular, greater auricular nerve as well as the stylohyoid (lateral) and posterior belly of the digastric (medial).

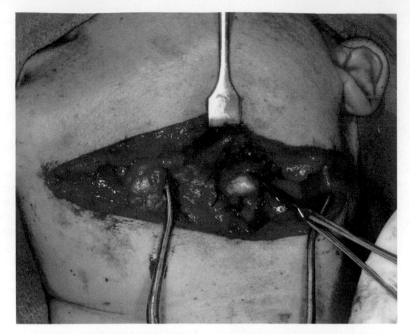

Fig. 28 The carotid body tumor is grasped.

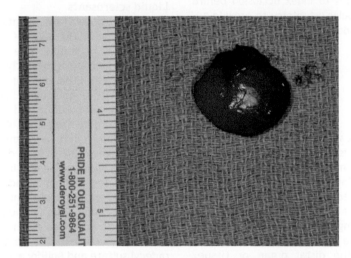

Fig. 29 Gross specimen of the carotid body tumor.

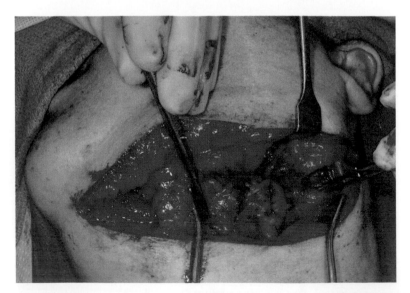

Fig. 30 Removal of tumor allows visualization of the common carotid, carotid bulb, internal and external carotid arteries, and hypoglossal nerve. Note also the sutures marking the transected stylohyoid (Prolene) and posterior belly of the digastric (silk) to facilitate reapproximation.

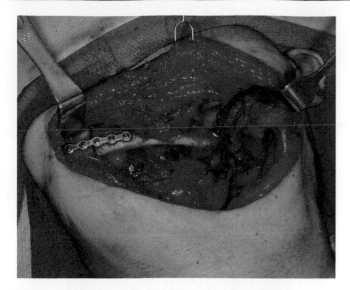

Fig. 31 Application of previously indexed bone plates ensures repeatable premorbid occlusion.

Thrombin

Thrombin is an enzyme that converts fibrinogen to fibrin, thus forming clots. It is most often used to aid thrombosis of post-procedure pseudoaneurysms. Pseudoaneurysms associated with masses that have a narrow neck can be treated with thrombin. It can be delivered via direct needle stick or catheter.

Gelfoam

Gelfoam is used as a powder embolic (10–100 μm diameter), in a slurry with contrast, or as small pledgets. Depending on its formulation, it will cause temporary vessel occlusion of either small or large vessels. Occlusion will last from days to a few weeks, but is unpredictable.

Coils

Coils come in a variety of sizes, shapes, metals (eg, steel-stiff, platinum-soft), and coatings (eg, thrombogenic coat) (see Figs. 19 and 20; Figs. 35 and 36). In addition, the coils have small fibers that provide a framework for platelet aggregation. This thrombosis provides relatively precise,

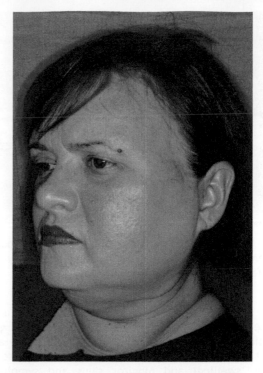

Fig. 32 The patient 4 months after surgery.

permanent, large-vessel occlusion at the level of the coil. Multiple coils are usually tightly packed together to create this desired effect. The Amplatzer Vascular Plug is a nitinol mesh device from 4 to 16 mm in diameter, which can be used in nontapering vessels to provide a scaffold for coils to create a precise vessel occlusion.

Percutaneous sclerotherapy

Percutaneous sclerotherapy is typically used for low-flow vascular malformations (either symptomatic or cosmetically problematic) (see Figs. 1–5). History and physical examination and preprocedure imaging determine the approach and embolic agent. Less involved lesions lend themselves well to

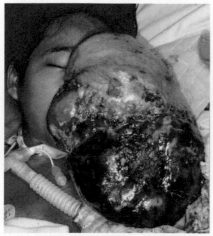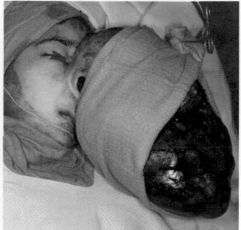

Fig. 33 (*Left*) A pediatric patient with a left facial mass. (*Right*) Significant ischemia 12 hours after select embolization of the collateral circulation. See Figs. 36 to 47 in the article by Webb and Ward elsewhere in this issue for case series.

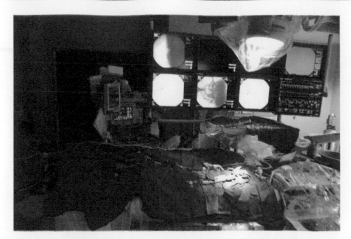

Fig. 34 View of the interventional radiology suite. The patient is under general anesthesia while traditional angiography is performed, facilitating preoperative select embolization.

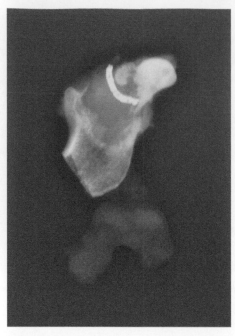

Fig. 36 Specimen radiograph showing a portion of the resected embolized internal maxillary artery (and associated coil).

moderate sedation. Extensive lesions often require general anesthesia (especially when using absolute ethanol) and an overnight inpatient stay to manage postprocedural sequelae (ie, pain, swelling) and monitor signs and symptoms of nontarget embolization. When performed in the angiography suite, the patient is induced, prepped, and draped, and a needle is placed into the malformation using ultrasound guidance. Contrast is then introduced into the malformation under fluoroscopy until it fills the lesion. The volume of contrast is noted, and absolute ethanol is injected under fluoroscopy at approximately one-half the volume of contrast. Multiple areas of the malformation can be targeted in a single setting; however, this increases the risk of nontarget complications. Complications occur 10% to 15% of the time, and most

commonly include skin necrosis or nerve/muscle injury. Only about 20% of patients will be completely treated in a single session.

Transarterial embolization

Percutaneous sclerotherapy injections would be difficult to control in patients with high-flow vascular malformations. As these lesions are arterialized, treatment options include a transarterial embolization or a percutaneous injection with intra-arterial balloon occlusion. Transarterial embolization is performed under moderate sedation in the angiography suite.

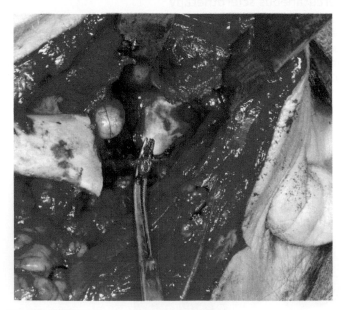

Fig. 35 The embolized internal maxillary artery was encountered during a left mandibular disarticulation segmental resection (pictured here with coil extruding). Mandibular fossa and articular eminence of the temporal bone, and the buccal fat pad, are in view. See Figs. 23 to 35 in the article by Webb and Ward elsewhere in this issue for case series.

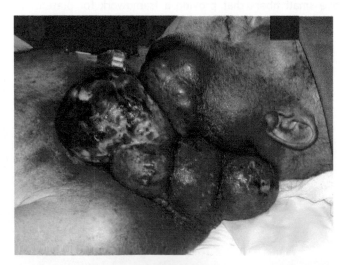

Fig. 37 A patient with large melanoma metastasis to the left supraclavicular region complicated by bleeding requiring transfusion. The lesion was deemed unresectable, and palliative embolization was requested.

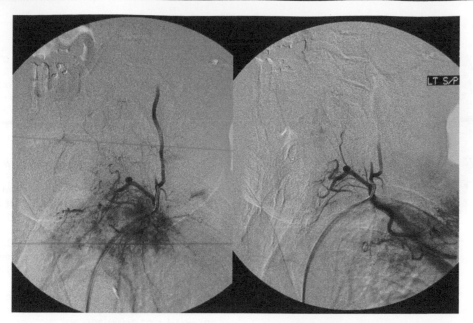

Fig. 38   (*Left*) Digital subtraction angiogram of lesion supplied by costoclavicular trunk. (*Right*) After particle embolization.

Catheters are advanced to the level of the feeding artery using fluoroscopy and embolization, performed with glue or particles depending on the nidus and the degree of flow. Sometimes combinations of embolic material are necessary (eg, coils in the setting of an AVF). Transarterial embolization can also be used to palliate symptoms associated with unresectable tumors (Figs. 37 and 38).

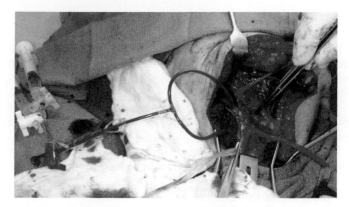

Fig. 40   An arteriotomy was performed from the common carotid extending cephalically to the distal aspect of the internal carotid artery. A Pruitt-Inahara shunt was then inserted, and the endarterectomy was completed under shunting.

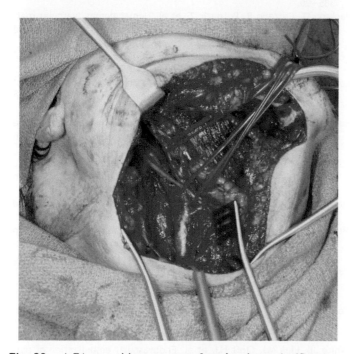

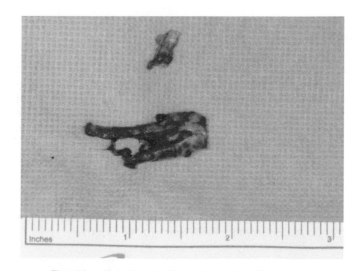

Fig. 39   A 74-year-old woman was found to have significant carotid stenosis extending above the angle of the mandible to within 2 cm of the skull base. Vascular surgeons considered the extensive atherosclerotic disease to be unapproachable by endovascular means secondary to extreme calcification. Typical access would not be sufficient to perform an endarterectomy. An Attia double mandibular osteotomy, shown here, provided the vascular surgeons with adequate access.

Fig. 41   Heavily calcified atherosclerotic plaque.

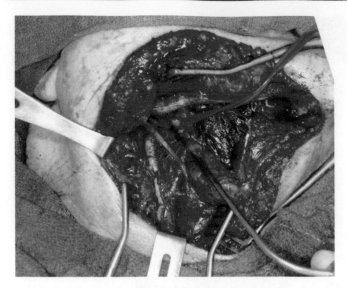

Fig. 42 After the endarterectomy was completed, a bovine pericardium patch was sutured in place.

Pearls

The key to good surgery is good access, and the key to good access is good surgery. This maxim is never more true than when dealing with vascular lesions—which demand unrestricted exposure (Figs. 39—42).

Hypervascular tumors or those known to have a high degree of blood loss during surgery may benefit from preoperative embolization.

If embolization is necessary, the embolic agent can be determined by using the following 3-question algorithm:

1. Is the vessel to be embolized large or small?
2. How long (temporally) is the vessel to remain occluded?
3. Is the tissue supplied by the vessel to remain viable after the embolization?

Surgery is usually performed the day after embolization, although some investigators suggest that resection can be delayed up to 8 days.

Summary

A coordinated, multidisciplinary approach to vascular anomalies of the neck will optimize patient outcomes. High-quality imaging, usually MRI, answers many of the clinical questions that arise before intervention. Vascular anomaly interventions range from oral medication, to image-guided definitive treatments, to combined preoperative embolization and surgery.

Supplementary data

Supplementary data related to this article can be found online at http://dx.doi.org/10.1016/j.exom.2011.11.001.

Further readings

Atkinson DS Jr, Ptak T. Neuroradiology case of the day. Am J Roentgenol 1999;173(3):804—12.

Barnes L, Eveson JW, Reichart P, et al, editors. World health organization classification of tumours. pathology and genetics of head and neck tumours. Lyon (France): IARC Press; 2005.

Buckmiller LM, Richter GT, Suen JY, et al. Diagnosis and management of hemangiomas and vascular malformations of the head and neck. Oral Dis 2010;16(5):405—18.

Callen J. Dermatology. 2nd edition. Spain: Mosby Elsevier; 2008. p. 1589—91, 1785—88.

Capatina C, Ntali G, Karavitaki N, et al. The management of head and neck paragangliomas. Endocr Relat Cancer 2013;20:R291—305.

Donnelly LF. Combined sonographic and fluoroscopic guidance: a modified technique for percutaneous sclerosis of low-flow vascular malformations. Am J Roentgenol 1999;173(3):655—7.

Donnelly LF. Vascular malformations and hemangiomas: a practical approach in a multidisciplinary clinic. Am J Roentgenol 2000;174(3):597—608.

Enjolras O. Classification and management of the various superficial vascular anomalies: hemangiomas and vascular malformations. J Dermatol 1997;24(11):701—10.

Fletcher CD, Unni KK, Mertens F, editors. World health organization classification of tumours. pathology and genetics of tumours of soft tissue and bone. Lyon (France): IARC Press; 2002.

Fletcher CD, Gustafson P, Rydholm A, et al, editors. World health organization classification of tumours. pathology and genetics of tumours of soft tissue and bone. Lyon (France): IARC Press; 2013.

Flors L, Leiva-Salinas C, Maged IM, et al. MR imaging of soft-tissue vascular malformations: diagnosis, classification, and therapy follow-up. Radiographics 2011;31(5):1321—40.

Gnepp DR, editor. Diagnostic surgical pathology of the head and neck. Philadelphia: Saunders Elsevier; 2009. p. 205—7, 233—37, 385—90.

Jackson IT, Carreño R, Potparic Z, et al. Hemangiomas, vascular malformations, and lymphovenous malformations: classification and methods of treatment. Plast Reconstr Surg 1993;91(7):1216—30.

Léauté-Labrèze C, Dumas de la Roque E, Hubiche T, et al. Propranolol for severe hemangioma of infancy. N Engl J Med 2008;358:2649—51.

Lowe LH, Marchant TC, Rivard DC, et al. Vascular malformations: classification and terminology the radiologist needs to know. Semin Roentgenol 2012;47(2):106—17.

Lubarsky M, Ray CE, Funaki B, et al. Embolization agents- which one should be used when? part 1: large-vessel embolization. Semin Intervent Radiol 2009;26(4):352—7.

Lubarsky M, Ray C, Funaki B, et al. Embolization agents- which one should be used when? part 2: small-vessel embolization. Semin Intervent Radiol 2010;27(1):99—104.

Marler JJ, Mulliken JB. Current management of hemangiomas and vascular malformations. Clin Plast Surg 2005;32(1):99—116.

Mulliken JB, Glowacki J. Hemangiomas and vascular malformations in infants and children: a classification based on endothelial characteristics. Plast Reconstr Surg 1982;69(3):412—22.

Pauw BK, Makek MS, Fisch U, et al. Preoperative embolization of paragangliomas (glomus tumors) of the head and neck- histopathologic and clinical features. Skull Base Surg 1993;3(1):37—44.

Perkins JA, Chen EY. Vascular anomalies of the head and neck. In: Flint P, editor. Cummings Otolaryngology — Head and Neck Surgery. 5th edition. Philadelphia: Mosby; 2010. p. 2822—34.

White JB, Link MJ, Cloft HJ, et al. Endovascular embolization of paragangliomas: a safe adjuvant to treatment. J Vasc Interv Neurol 2008;1(2):37—41.

Wushou A, Miao X, Shao Z. Treatment and outcome prognostic factors of head and neck hemangiopericytoma: a meta-analysis. Head Neck 2014. http://dx.doi.org/10.1002/hed.23812.

Soft Tissue Tumors of the Neck

David E. Webb, DDS [a], Brent B. Ward, DDS, MD [b],*

KEYWORDS

- Soft tissue tumors • Neck • Neoplasms • Biopsy

KEY POINTS

- Navigation within the complex structures of the neck, particularly where distortion exists, can be difficult; knowledge of normal anatomy, specific tumor characteristics, and ablative requirements must be applied to achieve successful treatment results.
- Advances in free tissue transfer have enabled the ablation of previously inoperable tumors.
- Given the variability of tumors in this region and associated resection requirements, imaging and preoperative biopsy should be routine for all but the smallest and most superficial tumors.
- Successful treatment should be assured with careful follow-up, including imaging when indicated.

General principles

Management of soft tissue tumors of the neck requires a great deal of expertise, both in terms of anatomic understanding, and surgical skill. Navigation within the complex structures of the neck, particularly where distortion exists, can be difficult. Knowledge of normal anatomy, specific tumor characteristics, and ablative requirements must be applied to achieve successful treatment results. This article reviews the treatment of soft tissue neoplasms of the neck.

Ideal functional and cosmetic outcomes are achieved by using surgical approaches that portend to optimal outcomes, sparing structures that can be reasonably spared, and reconstructing removed tissue whenever possible and appropriate. Advances in free tissue transfer have enabled the ablation of tumors that previously were considered inoperable because of size or location. Neck reconstruction using a large number of pedicled flaps remains an easy viable option with distinct advantages in select cases. Regardless of the method of reconstruction, clean surgical margins are paramount, and the overall ablative requirements must be the priority.

The ability to circumnavigate the neck is often important, given that in some lesions, utilization of a posterior approach is preferred. Surgeons comfortable with anterior approaches and anatomy may not intrinsically transfer this knowledge to the posterior neck when this is an uncommon operative field.

Given the variability of tumors in this region and associated resection requirements, imaging and preoperative biopsy should be routine for all but the smallest and most superficial tumors. Successful treatment should be assured with careful follow-up, including imaging when indicated.

Benign tumors

Lipoma

Lipomas overall represent the most common soft tissue tumor of the neck. Most lesions are located superficially in either the subcutaneous or dermal soft tissue (Figs. 1–8). Treatment of lipomas of the neck is determined by a number of factors, including location, size, involvement of critical adjacent structures, and reconstructive needs to optimize functional and cosmetic outcomes. Prior to biopsy, imaging studies are often helpful in understanding the full extent of the lesion. Although computed tomography (CT), ultrasound, and MRI are all used, MRI generally represents the ideal imaging modality. Preoperative biopsy is generally recommended unless tumors are small and classic in radiographic appearance. Lipomatous tumors have been divided by the World Health Organization into the following categories: ordinary lipoma, lipomatosis, lipomatosis of nerve, lipoblastoma/lipoblastomatosis, angiolipoma, myolipoma of soft tissue, chondroid lipoma, spindle cell/pleomorphic lipoma, and hibernoma. Treatment variations exist based on the various tumor types, another rationale advocating preoperative biopsy. For the purposes of this section, the focus will remain on ordinary lipoma.

Ordinary lipoma is the most common soft tissue tumor in adults, accounting for upwards of 30% to 50% of all soft tissue tumors of the body, with an incidence estimated at 0.5 to 1 case per 1000 population.[1] It occurs over a wide age range, but is most commonly diagnosed between the ages of 40 and 60 years, being somewhat rare in children. Approximately 10% present with multiple lipomas, which are often familial in nature and especially common in males. Approximately 13% to

The views expressed in this material are those of the authors, and do not reflect the official policy or position of the US Government, the Department of Defense, or the Department of the Air Force.

[a] Department of Oral and Maxillofacial Surgery, David Grant USAF Medical Center, 101 Bodin Circle/SGDD, Travis AFB, CA 94535, USA

[b] Oral/Head & Oncologic and Microvascular Reconstructive Surgery, Section of Oral and Maxillofacial Surgery, University of Michigan Hospitals, 1500 East Medical Center Drive, Ann Arbor, MI 48109, USA

* Corresponding author.

E-mail address: bward@umich.edu

http://dx.doi.org/10.1016/j.cxom.2014.11.002

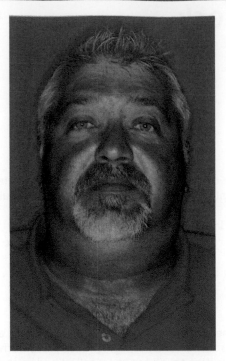

Fig. 1   46 year old man presented with a long-standing left neck mass. Patient concerned with recent growth of the mass and relatively new onset of pain.

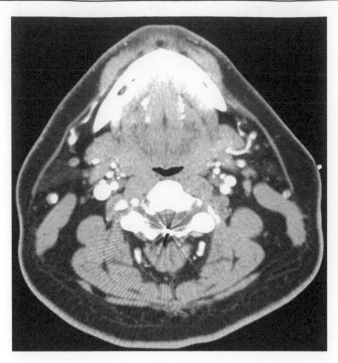

Fig. 3   Axial CT scan with contrast shows a mass superficial to the platysma whose density is similar to the adjacent subcutaneous fat.

17% of all lipomas are found in the head and neck region. They arise most frequently in the subcutaneous tissues and more rarely in deeper soft tissues. Most present as painless masses. Stable asymptomatic lesions less than 5 cm in size may be observed, although many are excised for cosmetic reasons. Simple excision is the treatment of choice, with a local recurrence rate of 4% to 5%.[2]

Peripheral nerve tumor (schwannoma or neurilemmoma)

Schwannomas are benign neoplasms of Schwann cell origin that surround peripheral nerves. Twenty-five percent to 45% of all schwannomas occur in the head and neck region extracranially.[3] They are most often solitary, well-encapsulated benign

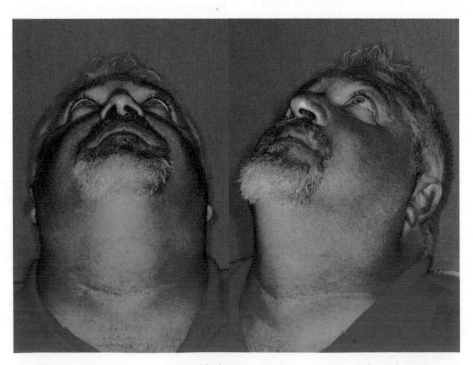

Fig. 2   Alternative views provide better visualization of the left neck mass.

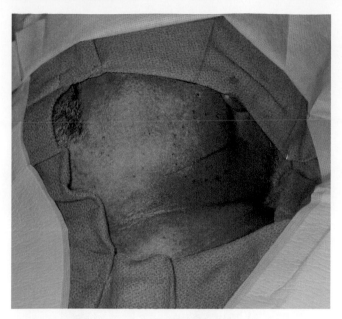

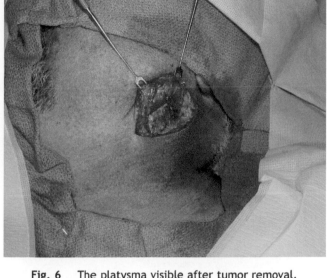

Fig. 6 The platysma visible after tumor removal.

Fig. 4 Proposed incision and delineation of left neck mass with marking pen. Also note the mandibular caudal border marking.

tumors running along the course of peripheral, cranial, or sympathetic nerves (Figs. 9–22). The rich neural supply of the neck gives many opportunities, with the vagus being the most common site. Schwannomas may be asymptomatic and found incidentally, or symptoms may include cough, hoarseness, dyspnea, dysphagia, tinnitus, Horner syndrome, and other neurologic deficits related to the involved nerve. Most often they present as a slowly growing neck mass. Schwannomas very rarely undergo malignant transformation. Even though less than 5% of cases arise in association with neurofibromatosis 2 (NF2), patients diagnosed with schwannoma should undergo a workup for possible NF2.[4] The mainstay of treatment is complete excision, resulting in a low rate of recurrence, but with concomitant postoperative neurologic deficits. Given the

morbidity associated with complete excision, some advocate a more conservative surgical approach involving intracapsular enucleation, thus decreasing the incidence of postoperative neurologic deficits from 100% to 31%. Yet others recommend close observation and reserve surgical intervention only for progressive or symptomatic tumors. Alternatively, when surgery is not an option, radiotherapy is utilized for tumor control.

Rhabdomyoma and leiomyoma

Rhabdomyomas are benign mesenchymal tumors with skeletal muscle differentiation. They are divided into extracardiac and intracardiac types, with the extracardiac type being extremely rare, but with a propensity for the head and neck. Fifteen percent of patients with extracardiac rhabdomyoma present with multifocal disease.[5] Extracardiac rhabdomyomas may further be divided into adult, fetal, genital, and rhabdomyomatous mesenchymal hamartoma. Adult type has a mean age of occurrence of 60, with males more frequently affected. When presenting as a mass in the neck, the most common muscles involved include the strap and sternocleidomastoid muscles. Treatment of these lesions is surgical excision. Recurrence rates may be as high as 42% and have been

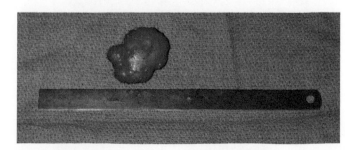

Fig. 7 Gross specimen measuring 4 × 3 cm. Serial sectioning of the homogenous tan—yellow specimen confirmed a diagnosis of lipoma.

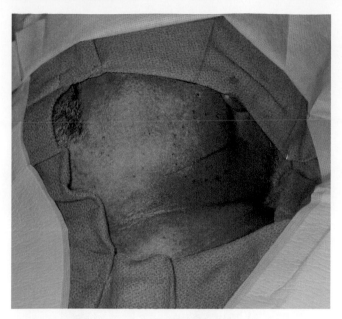

Fig. 5 Cirumferential pericapsular dissection allowed the mass to herniate outward.

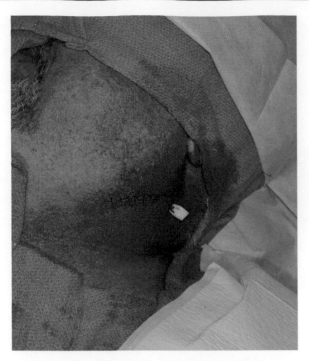

Fig. 8 Final closure of the neck with a 0.25 inch Penrose drain in place.

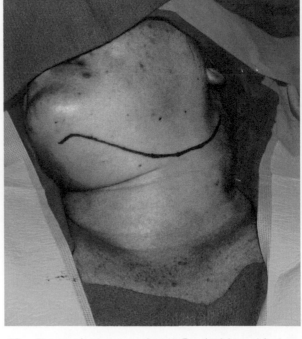

Fig. 10 Proposed upper member McFee incision with dots representing the mandibular caudal border.

reported as late as 35 years after initial treatment. It is felt that these failures are likely caused by either incomplete excision or secondary to the multifocality of the disease.

Leiomyoma is a benign soft-tissue neoplasm arising from smooth muscle. A hereditary form causing multiple lesions exists. Occurrence in the head and neck is extremely rare (1%) given the fact that smooth muscle in this region is lacking.

Leiomyomas are usually solitary, rounded, well-demarcated masses. Histopathological analysis and immunochemical analysis are important for distinction between this lesion and its malignant counterpart of leiomyosarcoma. Surgical excision is the treatment of choice, with recurrence being extremely rare.[6]

Malignant tumors

Each of the benign tumors previously reviewed have malignant counterparts. Recognizing the great variability and the atlas nature of this text, the authors' focus here will include only a few soft tissue sarcomas of the neck with some overriding principles of management. The authors note that

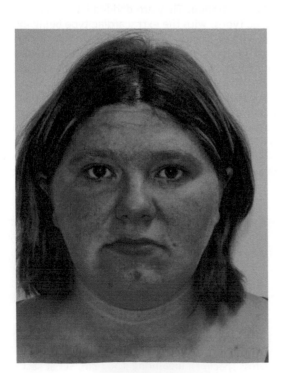

Fig. 9 29 year old woman with a 2-month history of vertigo, headaches, fever, and syncopal episodes ×2.

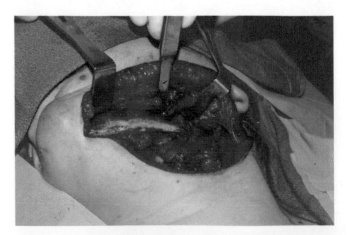

Fig. 11 Preparing the mandible for the Attia double osteotomy by preserving cephalic periosteum as well as the mental branch of the inferior alveolar nerve.

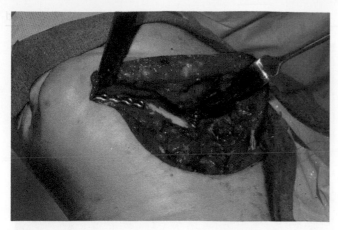

Fig. 12 Indexing osseous segments with bone plates prior to osteotomies.

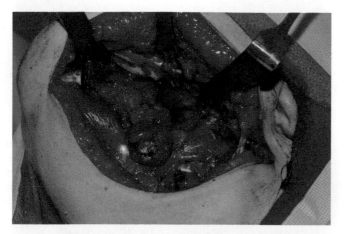

Fig. 13 Osteotomized mandible allows for cephalic rotation and direct access to the left parapharyngeal space tumor.

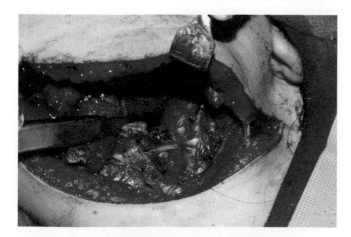

Fig. 14 Left parapharygneal tumor immediately adjacent to carotid artery. Note the relationship of the hypoglossal nerve and the carotid artery. Greater auricular nerve preserved at lateral extent of incision overlying the sternocleidomastoid muscle. Intentional transection of the stylohoid and posterior digastric muscles has been marked with sutures to facilitate reapproximation after tumor removal.

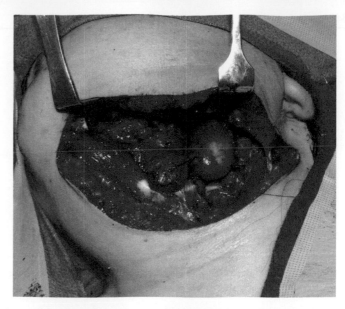

Fig. 15 The encapsulated tumor has been mobilized and now lies superficially within the parapharyngeal space.

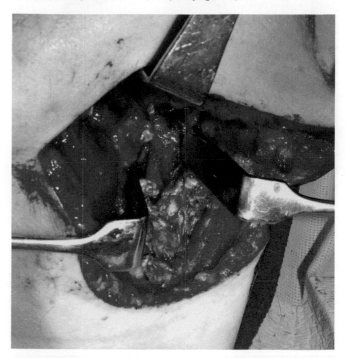

Fig. 16 Tumor removal allows direct visualization of the internal carotid artery as seen between the opposing Obwegeser retractors.

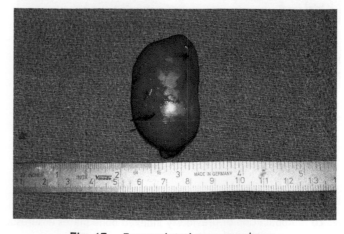

Fig. 17 Encapsulated gross specimen.

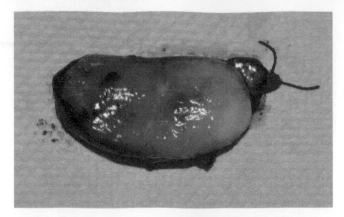

Fig. 18 Gross specimen inked and bisected. Microscopy revealed well-developed Verocay bodies with S-100 immunostain confirming neural origin consistent with schwannoma.

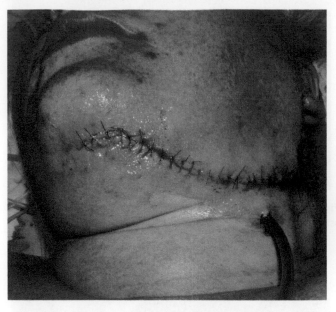

Fig. 21 Final closure with 7 mm flat Bard drain in place.

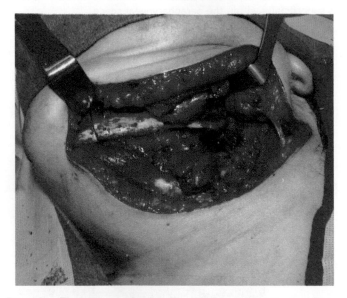

Fig. 19 The osteotomized segments are realigned after tumor removal.

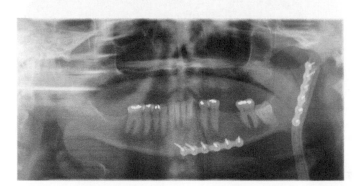

Fig. 22 Postoperative radiograph showing hardware and drain in left parapharygneal space.

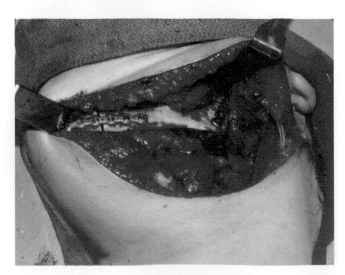

Fig. 20 Application of previously indexed bone plates ensures a postoperative unaltered occlusion.

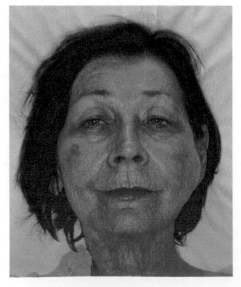

Fig. 23 68-year-old woman presented with a recent onset of left facial swelling and pain. Fine needle aspiration biopsy (FNAB) favored a poorly differentiated carcinoma.

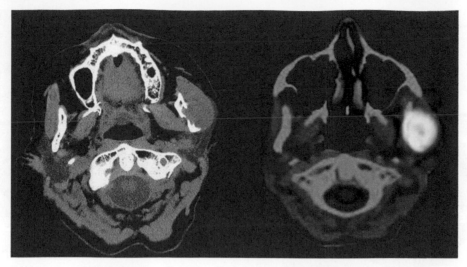

Fig. 24 Preoperative imaging identified a hypermetabolic left mandibular mass intimately associated with the left internal maxillary artery.

recommendations for specific tumor types exist and are beyond the scope of this article.

Overall, sarcomas are rare malignancies accounting for less than 1% of all tumors of the body and are especially uncommon in the head and neck except in the pediatric population.[7,8] A review of experience from the MD Anderson head and neck service over 30 years revealed only 802 patients out of over 30,000 total cancer diagnoses.[9] In most reports, sarcomas of the head and neck represent 4% to 10% of all adult sarcomas.[10] Sarcomas are classified by tissue of origin, histologic grade, and anatomic subsite, with 80% of head and neck sarcomas derived from soft tissue. Histologic grading is particularly important in guiding management decisions, particularly as it relates to the

use of neoadjuvant and adjuvant therapies (radiation, chemotherapy, and combined modalities). Individualized grading systems exist for the various subtypes of sarcoma.

Malignant fibrous histiocytoma

Malignant fibrous histiocytoma (MFH) represents approximately 5% of all soft tissue sarcomas in adults, with less than 10% in the head and neck (Figs. 23–35).[11] These lesions, like other sarcomas, can occur in patients with a history of radiation exposure, which portends a poorer prognosis. The mass is usually painless and subcutaneous and seldom presents with regional or distant metastasis. Treatment is wide local excision for

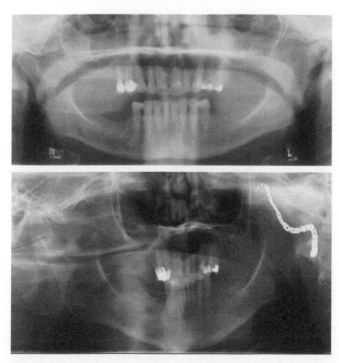

Fig. 25 Presurgical panoramic radiographs. Postcoil embolization of the internal maxillary artery below.

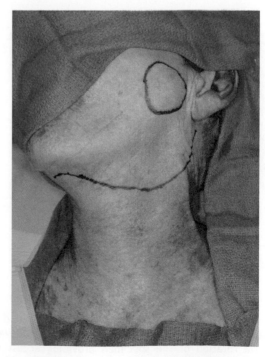

Fig. 26 Proposed incision and tumor location delineated.

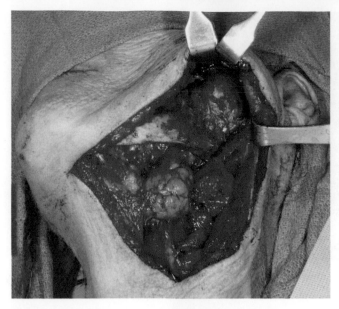

Fig. 27 Surgical approach providing adequate access for resection. Coil embolization of the left internal maxillary artery was performed 3 days prior to resection.

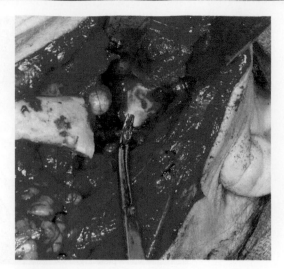

Fig. 29 The embolized internal maxillary artery was encountered pictured here with coil extruding. Mandibular fossa and articular eminence of the temporal bone in addition to the buccal fat pad in view.

negative margins, and elective cervical lymphadenectomy is unnecessary given its low regional metastatic potential. Positive margins at the time of surgery are associated with decreased local control and increased incidence of distant disease. Postoperative radiotherapy is recommended for unresectable lesions or those with close or positive margins and may be beneficial even when wide margins have been achieved. Adjuvant chemotherapy may or may not be beneficial. Overall 5-year survival rates for MFH are 40% in larger series but

range from 19% to 75% in smaller reports. Approximately 20% of patients experience local recurrence, with most deaths related to distant disease, particularly arising in the lungs. Smaller lesions (< 5 cm), low grade status, negative margins, and certain histologic subtypes (myxoid and angiomatoid) result in a better prognosis.

Rhabdomyosarcoma

Rhabdomyosarcoma is a common sarcoma in the pediatric population (Figs. 36—47) but quite rare in adults, particularly

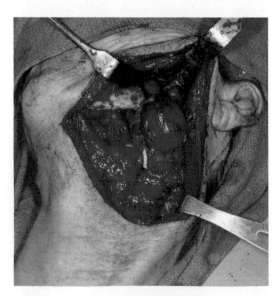

Fig. 28 En bloc resection was accomplished via a left disarticulation segmental resection. The distal osteotomy allowed for caudolateral rotation of the specimen providing access to the remaining medial and cephalic margins.

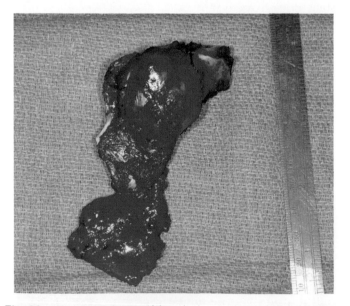

Fig. 30 Gross specimen. Although the positron emission tomography CT scan failed to demonstrate abnormal fluorodeoxyglucose (FDG) avidity in cervical lymph nodes, a limited cervical lymphadenectomy was performed based on intraoperative suspicion. All lymph nodes were negative for microscopic disease.

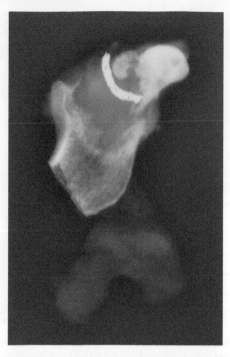

Fig. 31 Specimen radiograph showing a portion of the resected embolized internal maxillary artery (and associated coil).

as it pertains to the neck. Rhabdomyosarcomas present as 1 of 4 defined subtypes (embryonal, alveolar, botryoidal, or pleomorphic). In adults, alveolar and pleomorphic are most common, particularly since the percentage of alveolar subtype increases with age. Although a great deal of experience has been gleaned from the pediatric population, it is unclear if success there translates to the adult population.[12,13] Careful workup for distant metastasis is important in rhabdomyosarcoma given the propensity for individuals to harbor distant disease on presentation. Classification is of clinical

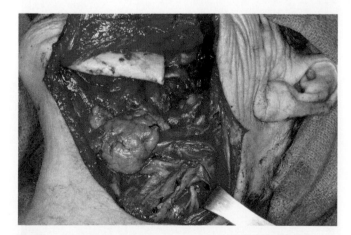

Fig. 32 Postresection photograph shows an intact lingual nerve and anterior and posterior digastric muscles with overlying submandibular gland. Also visible is the stylohyoid muscle, hypoglossal nerve, internal jugular vein (with ligated branches), and a portion of the ansa cervicalis.

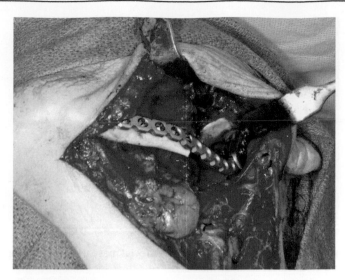

Fig. 33 Immediate reconstruction performed with a reconstruction plate and affixed condylar prosthesis.

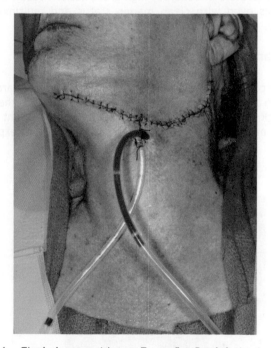

Fig. 34 Final closure with two 7 mm flat Bard drains in place.

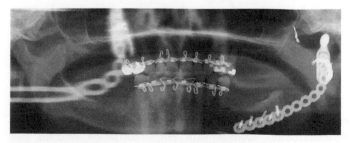

Fig. 35 Postoperative radiograph. Note the coil discontinuity of the previously embolized left internal maxillary artery.

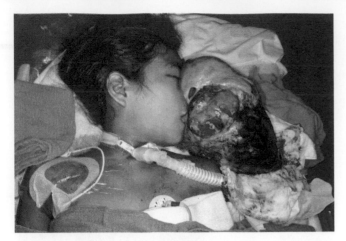

Fig. 36 Pediatric patient with a left facial mass. Note the diaper used to enclose/conceal the mass.

relevance given that alveolar subtypes are particularly incurable. Regardless of subtype, high-grade lesions result in poor prognosis even with clean margin status and multimodality therapy.

Fibrosarcoma

Fibrosarcoma is one of the more common soft tissue sarcomas but with a small number (approximately 5%) arising in the head and neck (Figs. 48–60). Fibrosarcomas generally present in the fourth and fifth decades, with prior radiation exposure

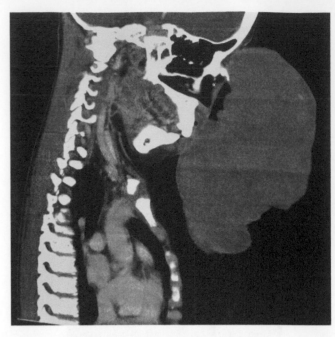

Fig. 38 Sagittal Computed Tomography Angiography (CTA) demonstrating a massive pedunculated lesion extending from orbit to maxilla.

documented in upwards of 10% of cases. It usually presents as a firm painless neck mass. Approximately 10% of patients with fibrosarcoma report a history of radiation exposure. Wide surgical excision is the mainstay of therapy given that local recurrence is particularly problematic and frequently the eventual cause of death. Tumor grade is the most important prognostic factor followed by tumor size and margin status. Adjuvant radiation and chemotherapy are employed,

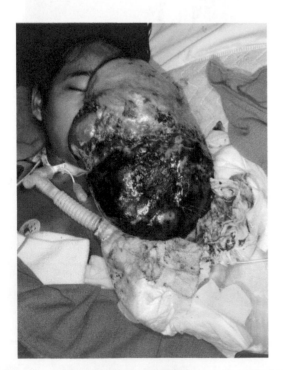

Fig. 37 An additional view provided to compare baseline ischemia/tissue necrosis with postembolization necrosis (see Fig. 41). Note the tracheotomy and central line access were accomplished prior to select embolization.

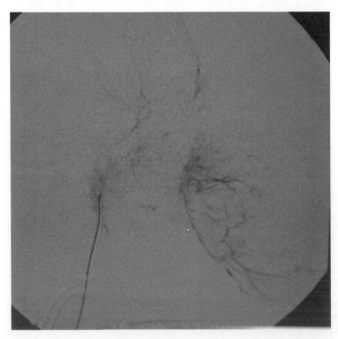

Fig. 39 Selected external carotid angiogram in the parenchymal phase showing extensive collateral circulation to the mass.

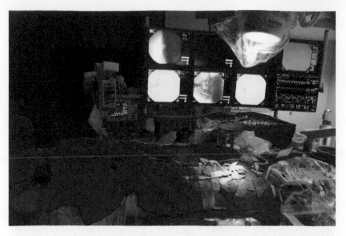

Fig. 40 View of the interventional radiology suite. Patient under general anesthesia while traditional angiography is performed, facilitating preoperative select embolization.

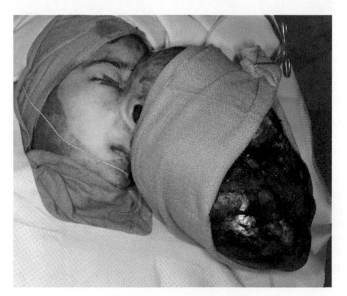

Fig. 41 Note the significant ischemia/necrosis 12 hours after select embolization of the collateral circulation. This photograph was obtained immediately prior to resection.

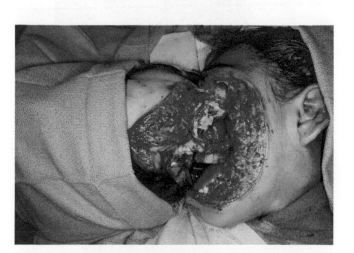

Fig. 42 Tumor ablation consisted of left orbital exenteration, left rhinectomy, left partial maxillectomy, left partial parotidectomy, and partial upper/lower lip resections with left facial nerve integrity monitoring. See Video 1 in this issue's Vascular Anomalies of the Neck article by Webb and colleagues to appreciate the flammable nature of Onyx (a liquid adhesive embolic material).

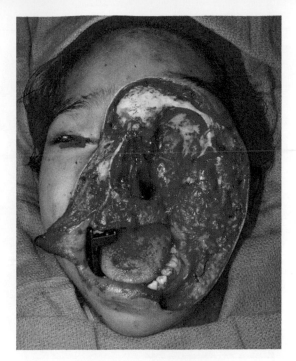

Fig. 43 Postablative defect.

particularly for high-grade and larger tumors. As with other sarcomas, high-grade status results in poorer prognosis. Distant metastasis is problematic for this tumor, reported as 34% at 1 year, 52% at 2 years, and 63% at 5 years, with late metastasis reported up to 22 years after removal of primary disease. When negative margins can be achieved, fibrosarcoma has a relatively favorable survival rate compared with other neck sarcomas. Five-year survival ranges from 63% to 82%, with disease-free survival ranging from 32% to 57%.

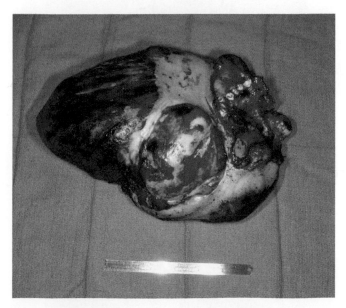

Fig. 44 Gross specimen. Microscopic analysis yielded a final diagnosis of embryonal rhabdomyosarcoma.

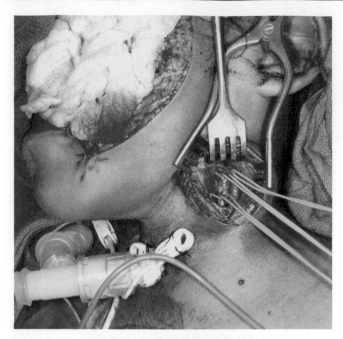

Fig. 45   Preparation of recipient vessels for free tissue transfer.

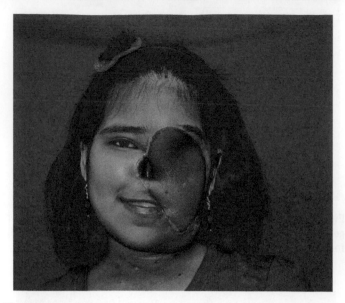

Fig. 47   Healed free flap just prior to maxillofacial prosthesis fabrication.

Neurogenic sarcoma

Neurogenic sarcoma includes terminology encompassing malignant peripheral nerve sheath tumor, malignant schwannoma, malignant neurofibroma, and neurofibrosarcoma. These are relatively rare tumors, with only 5% of overall soft tissue sarcomas, but 20% of them occur in the head and neck, indicative of the rich neural supply in the region. Half of all lesions are associated with neurofibromatosis type I (NF1).

Sporadic cases occur in the fourth to sixth decades, with equal sex distribution. The most common presentation is a painless enlarging neck mass, although neuropathy may also be a symptom. Distinguishing these lesions from other histologic types is often challenging. Neurogenic sarcomas are classified as low-, intermediate-, or high-grade lesions. Wide excision with negative margins is key, as propensity for local recurrence is high. Radiation therapy has been utilized in the adjuvant setting, while the role of chemotherapy remains in question. Distant metastasis is relatively common, occurring in approximately 30% of patients.

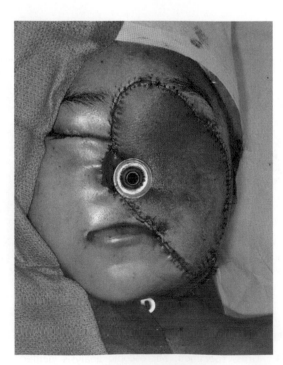

Fig. 46   Nasopharyngeal airway in place after free flap inset.

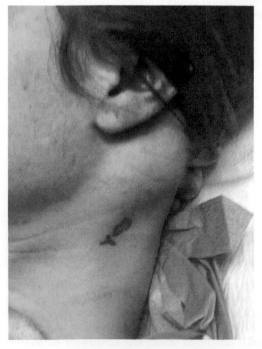

Fig. 48   23-year-old woman with left posterior neck mass.

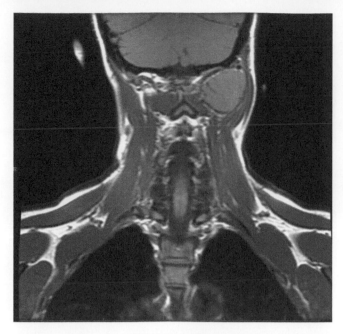

Fig. 49 MRI of posterior neck mass.

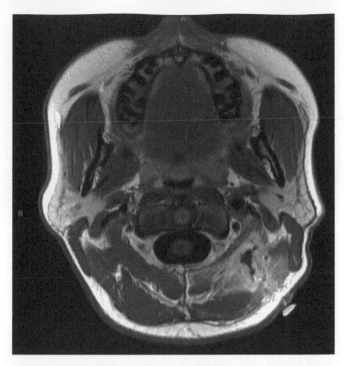

Fig. 51 Postoperative MRI with residual lesion versus postoperative changes.

Leiomyosarcoma

Leiomyosarcomas are thought to arise from smooth muscle or pluripotential, undifferentiated mesenchymal cells. They are the least common head and neck sarcomas, with the neck more commonly affected. Patients are generally in the fifth or sixth decades of life without sex predilection. Wide excision is the treatment of choice for these lesions, which are high grade, recur frequently, and demonstrate propensity for distant metastasis leading to consideration for adjuvant radiation and chemotherapy.

Dermatofibrosarcoma protuberans

Dermatofibrosarcoma protuberans (DFSP) is a low-grade cutaneous malignancy representing only 4% to 10% of all head and neck sarcomas. Men are more frequently affected, and the mean age is 31 years. The scalp is the most common site, but lesions throughout the neck occur with some frequency. Tumors appear as raised, painless nodules or plaques, often with reddish and bluish hue. Most lesions initially exhibit a slow radial growth pattern, but a rapid vertical (exophytic) phase ensues. Slow growth commonly leads to delayed diagnosis as well as misdiagnosis. Simple surgical excision leads to recurrence in approximately 50% of cases; therefore wide surgical

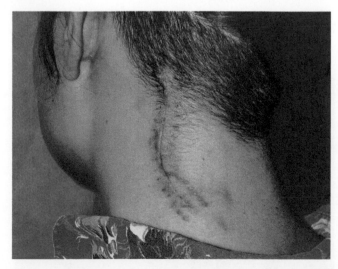

Fig. 50 Presentation on referral to secondary surgeon status after excision of the mass. Final pathology revealed high-grade myxofibrosarcoma with positive margins.

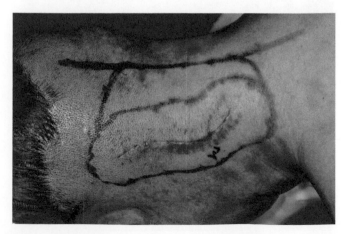

Fig. 52 Planned access with 2 cm margins and midline access for combined case with neurosurgery.

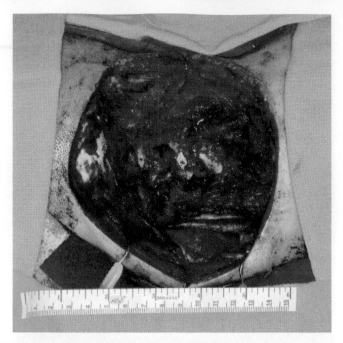

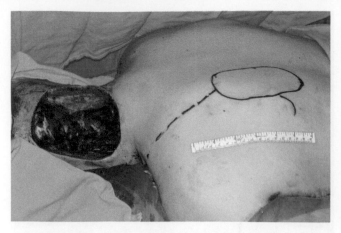

Fig. 55   Planned lower island trapezius flap.

Fig. 53   Surgical defect with protection of vertebral artery, internal jugular vein, and spinal accessory nerve.

excision of the primary lesion is the treatment of choice, with reconstruction after confirmation of negative margins.[14] Metastasis is extremely rare; therefore negative margins are the main indicator of survival. Radiation therapy has been employed when negative margins cannot be obtained.

Liposarcoma

Liposarcomas account for 35% to 45% of all soft tissue sarcomas, one of the most common sarcomas of adults. Liposarcoma of the head and neck is more rare, accounting for 2% to 9% of soft tissue

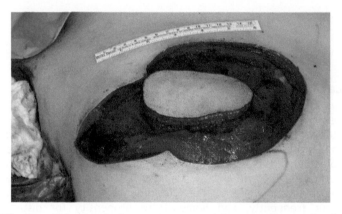

Fig. 56   Skin island of myocutaneous axial pattern flap outlined.

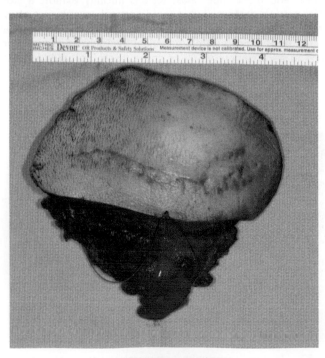

Fig. 54   Surgical specimen.

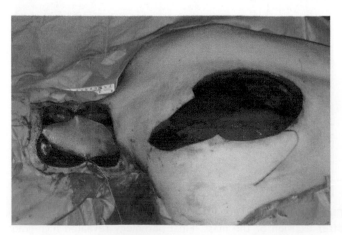

Fig. 57   Flap raised and tunneled to defect site.

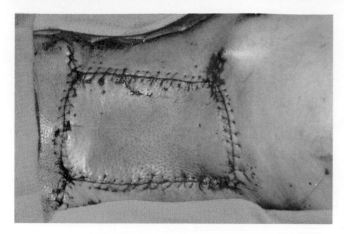

Fig. 58 Surgical site closure.

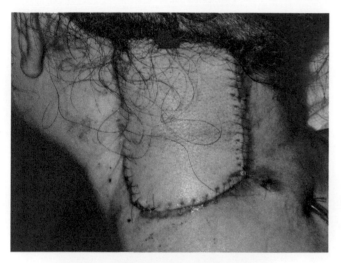

Fig. 59 Early postoperative appearance.

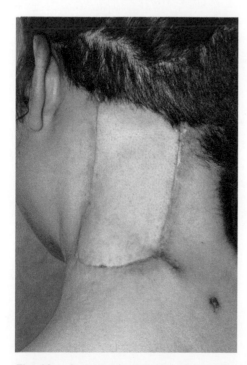

Fig. 60 One month postoperative result.

sarcomas in this body location. Liposarcomas have been divided into well-differentiated, myxoid, round-cell, pleomorphic, and mixed-type and not-otherwise-specified liposarcomas. Histologic grade is a primary determinate of survival, with pleomorphic and round-cell being considered as high-grade tumors. The mainstay of treatment for liposarcomas of the neck is wide surgical excision with generous clean margins. Achieving margins of this magnitude in the head and neck is always complex and often not possible. Regardless, a clean surgical margin is the primary determinant of survival. Adjuvant radiation therapy often follows surgery for enhancement of local control, although an overall survival benefit has not been documented. Liposarcomas do have a better prognosis overall than other soft tissue sarcomas of the head and neck. Treatment failures occur both locally and distantly, at rates of 50% to 80% and 10% to 15% respectively. As expected, survival for high-grade tumors is decreased compared with low-grade tumors. Multivariate analysis has demonstrated young age as a positive prognostic indicator with high-grade, salivary gland and pharyngeal involvement as negative indicators of survival.[15]

References

1. de Bree E, Karatzanis A, Hunt J, et al. Lipomatous tumours of the head and neck: a spectrum of biological behavior. Eur Arch Otorhinolaryngol 2014 [Epub ahead of print].
2. Myhre-Jensen O. A consecutive 7-year series of 1331benign soft tissue tumours. Clinicopathologic data. Comparison with sarcomas. Acta Orthop Scand 1981;52:287–93.
3. Yasumatsu R, Nakashima T, Miyazaki R, et al. Diagnosis and management of extracranial head and neck schwannomas: a review of 27 cases. Int J Otolaryngol 2013;2013:973045. http://dx.doi.org/10.1155/2013/973045.
4. Huq A, Kentwell M, Tirimacco A, et al. Vestibular schwannoma in a patient with neurofibromatosis type 1: clinical report and literature review. Fam Cancer 2014 [Epub ahead of print].
5. de Trey LA, Schmid S, Huber G. Multifocal adult rhabdomyoma of the head and neck manifestation in 7 locations and review of the literature. Case Rep Otolaryngol 2013;2013:758416. http://dx.doi.org/10.1155/2013/758416.
6. Veeresh M, Sudhakara M, Girish G, et al. Leiomyoma: a rare tumor in the head and neck and oral cavity: report of 3 cases with review. J Oral Maxillofac Pathol 2013;17(2):281–7.
7. O'Neill JP, Bilsky MH, Kraus D. Head and neck sarcomas: epidemiology, pathology, and management. Neurosurg Clin N Am 2013; 24(1):67–78.
8. Brockstein B. Management of sarcomas of the head and neck. Curr Oncol Rep 2004;6(4):321–7.
9. Potter BO, Sturgis EM. Sarcomas of the head and neck. Surg Oncol Clin N Am 2003;12(2):379–417.
10. Peng KA, Grogan T, Wang MB. Head and Neck Sarcomas: analysis of the SEER database. Otolaryngol Head Neck Surg 2014;151(4): 627–33. http://dx.doi.org/10.1177/0194599814545747.
11. Hardison SA, Davis PL 3rd, Browne JD. Malignant fibrous histiocytoma of the head and neck: a case series. Am J Otolaryngol 2013; 34(1):10–5.
12. Wu Y, Li C, Zhong Y, et al. Head and neck rhabdomyosarcoma in adults. J Craniofac Surg 2014;25(3):922–5.
13. Huber GF, Matthews TW, Dort JC. Radiation-induced soft tissue sarcomas of the head and neck. Soft-tissue sarcomas of the head and neck: a retrospective analysis of the Alberta experience 1974 to 1999. Laryngoscope 2006;116(5):780–5.
14. Goldberg C, Hoang D, McRae M, et al. A strategy for the successful management of dermatofibrosarcoma protuberans. Ann Plast Surg 2013 [Epub ahead of print].
15. Golledge J, Fisher C, Rhys-Evans PH. Head and neck liposarcoma. Cancer 1995;76:1051–8.

Metastatic Neck Disease

Melvyn S. Yeoh, DMD, MD*, Ryan J. Smart, DMD, MD,
Ghali E. Ghali, DDS, MD

KEYWORDS

- Neck mass • Metastatic neck disease • Fine needle aspiration (FNA) • Neck mass with unknown primary malignancy
- Malignancy • Cancer

KEY POINTS

- The differential diagnosis for neck masses is broad and can be tailored based on a thorough history and physical examination as well as by patient age.
- New neck masses in adult patients should be considered malignant until proven otherwise.
- Malignant neck masses are commonly painless with most patients developing symptoms from the primary tumor location.
- Diagnostic adjuncts in the workup for metastatic neck disease include CT and PET/CT imaging, MRI, ultrasound, and fine-needle aspiration biopsy.
- Metastatic neck masses are commonly secondary to oral, oropharyngeal, and nasopharyngeal carcinomas; less prevalent are metastases from other malignancies.

Introduction

The presence of metastatic neck disease in patients with head and neck cancer has a tremendous impact on the prognosis of these patients. Patients with head and neck cancer with tumors localized at the primary site without metastasis to the neck have an excellent prognosis with treatment. Although in patients with dissemination to regional cervical lymph nodes, the probability of a 5-year survival, regardless of treatment received, reduces their survival rate by 50%. Even with increased public education and awareness, a large number of patients still present with advanced disease at the time of diagnosis. The American Cancer Society has found that about 40% of the patients with squamous cell carcinoma of the upper aerodigestive tract have clinically evident regional metastatic disease during their initial presentation. Thus, the understanding of the anatomy, dissemination of disease, and treatment of the metastatic neck disease is vital when managing patients with head and neck cancers.

Anatomy of the cervical lymphatics

The lymphatic drainage in the neck can be divided into the central neck compartment and the lateral compartment. Central compartment lymph nodes include lymph nodes in the prelaryngeal, pretracheal, paratracheal, and tracheoesophageal groove. The pretracheal lymph node, also known as the Delphian lymph node, provides drainage from the larynx and thyroid gland. The lymph nodes in the prelaryngeal,

paratracheal, and tracheoesophageal groove also provide drainage for the thyroid gland as well as the hypopharynx, subglottic larynx, and cervical esophagus. Boundaries of the central compartment of the neck are demarcated by the hyoid bone superiorly, the innominate artery inferiorly, and the medial borders of the carotid sheath laterally. Cervical lymph nodes in the lateral aspect of the neck primarily drain the mucosa of the upper aerodigestive tract.

The lateral neck is divided into the anterior triangle and the posterior triangle. Lymph nodes in the anterior triangle of the lateral neck include the submental, prevascular facial, and submandibular lymph node chains located in the submental and submandibular triangles of the neck. The deep jugular lymph nodes include the jugulodigastric, jugulo-omohyoid, and supraclavicular group of lymph nodes adjacent to the internal jugular vein (IJV). Cervical lymph nodes located in the posterior triangle of the neck include the accessory chain of lymph nodes located along the spinal accessory nerve and transverse cervical chain of lymph nodes in the floor of the posterior neck. The base of the anterior triangle of the lateral neck lies along the inferior border of the mandible with its peak at the sternoclavicular joint. The lateral margin is the sternocleidomastoid, while the central neck structures border medially. The posterior triangle of the lateral neck is bounded by the posterior border of the sternocleidomastoid muscle (SCM) anteriorly, anterior border of the trapezius muscle posteriorly, and the clavicle inferiorly.

The Memorial Sloan-Kettering Cancer Center leveling system of lymph nodes provides an orderly manner of describing the location of cervical lymph nodes between the clinician and pathologist (Fig. 1). This system divides the lateral neck into 5 levels or nodal groups and the central neck into 2 levels. Level I lymph nodes are located superior to the hyoid bone and the digastric muscle to the inferior border of the mandible. They can be further divided into the submental (level IA) and

Department of Oral and Maxillofacial Surgery, LSU Health Sciences Center, Shreveport, LA, USA

* Corresponding author.
E-mail address: myeoh@lsuhsc.edu

Atlas Oral Maxillofacial Surg Clin N Am 23 (2015) 95–104
1061-3315/15/$ - see front matter © 2015 Elsevier Inc. All rights reserved.
http://dx.doi.org/10.1016/j.cxom.2014.10.003

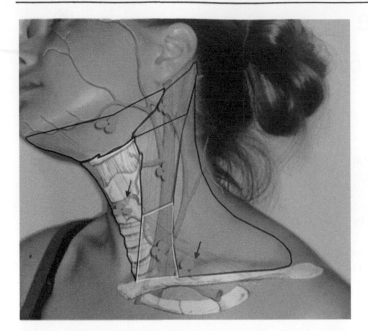

Fig. 1 Photograph demonstrating the levels of the neck with bony, muscular, and visceral landmarks. Level 1 is outlined in lavender; level 2 is outlined in red; level 3 is outlined in green; level 4 is outlined in yellow; level 5 is outlined in black; and level 6 is outlined in navy. The lymph nodes seen in these levels are shown as green ovals. Pretracheal "Delphian" node (*black arrow*). "Virchow" node (*red arrow*) at the junction of the left lymphatic duct and subclavian vein (lymphatic duct not shown).

submandibular (level IB) groups. Submental group lymph nodes are located anterior to the anterior belly of the digastric muscle and cephalad to the hyoid bone up to the inferior border of the mandible. Lymph nodes located posterior to the anterior belly of the digastric muscle and superior to the anterior and posterior bellies of the digastric muscle up to the inferior border of the mandible are the submandibular group. Level II lymph nodes are located around the upper portion of the IJV and the upper portion of the spinal accessory nerve extending from the base of the skull downwards to the bifurcation of the carotid artery. Level III lymph nodes are around the middle portion of the IJV starting from the inferior border of level II extending downwards to the omohyoid muscle. Level IV lymph nodes are the lower portion of the IJV extending from the inferior border of level III downwards to the clavicle. The anterior and posterior borders of level II, III, and IV are the lateral limit of the sternohyoid muscle and the posterior border of the SCM, respectively. The posterior triangle group or level IV is bound by the triangle formed by the clavicle, posterior border of the SCM, and the anterior border of the trapezius muscle (see Fig. 1). The central compartment of the neck is broken down into level VI and VII. Level VI lymph nodes are from the hyoid bone to the suprasternal notch and between the medial borders of the carotid sheath. Level VII, the superior mediastinal group, are the lymph nodes located in the anterior mediastinum extending from the innominate artery inferiorly to the suprasternal notch.

Risk of nodal metastases

Malignancies of the head and neck region frequently involve the cervical lymphatics. Involvement of the regional

lymphatics depends on various factors, such as type of primary tumor, location of primary tumor, T stage, and histomorphologic features of the primary tumor. Squamous cell carcinoma of the upper digestive tract is the most common type of cancer to metastasize to the cervical lymphatics. The risk of nodal metastasis of squamous cell carcinoma of the upper aerodigestive tract varies with location of the primary tumor. The risk increases as one progresses from anterior to posterior within the upper aerodigestive tract: lips, oral cavity, oropharynx, and hypopharynx. In primary tumors of the pharynx and larynx, the risk of regional nodal metastasis increases as one progresses from the center to the periphery. Thus, the risk of metastasis increases as one moves from the vocal cords, being the lowest risk, to the false vocal cords, aryepiglottic fold, pyriform sinus, and pharyngeal wall, being the highest risk. Certain primary sites can also have an increased risk of nodal metastases compared with the other primary sites in the same region. For example, in the oral cavity, squamous cell carcinoma of the floor of the mouth has a higher risk compared with the hard palate. The T stage reflects the tumor burden of the primary tumor, and an increasing T stage correlates with a higher risk of cervical metastasis.[1]

Certain histomorphologic features of the primary tumor also increase the risk of nodal metastasis. Poorly differentiated carcinomas have a higher risk compared with well-differentiated carcinomas. Endophytic tumors have also been noted to be more inclined to metastasize compared with exophytic tumors. The tumor thickness in carcinoma of the floor of the mouth and tongue has been well documented to relate to the risk of nodal metastases. In practice, if the risk of occult metastases exceeds 15%, then elective treatment of regional lymph nodes is recommended because it can affect the prognosis of the patient.

Other malignancies of the head and neck region include carcinomas of salivary origin, skin cancers, and thyroid cancers. Metastasis to the cervical lymph nodes from carcinomas of salivary origin tend to be low (<20%), but high-stage (T3 and T4) and high-grade (poorly differentiated) tumors warrant elective treatment of the neck. The risk of neck metastasis from cutaneous cancers of the head and neck is variable. Basal cell carcinomas have a very low risk of metastasis. Small squamous cell carcinomas (<2 cm) of the skin of the head and neck have a very low risk of nodal metastasis, but as the size increases, so does the risk. However, cutaneous melanoma has a predictably high risk of nodal metastasis with increasing thickness and size of the primary tumor. Thus, one can justify the need for elective treatment of the regional lymph nodes for thicker melanomas. Sentinel node mapping has become an available procedure in patients with head and neck cancers of various types but has become particularly popular in patients with cutaneous head and neck melanomas.[2] Regional dissemination of metastasis is quite high in thyroid cancer but elective dissection of regional lymph nodes is not recommended in well-differentiated thyroid carcinomas (papillary and follicular), because it generally does not change the prognosis.

Cervical metastasis can also be the result of dissemination from primary tumors not in the head and neck region. Masses in the supraclavicular area raise suspicion for primary lung lesion metastasis as well as abdominal malignancies, especially gastric cancer. Virchow node, named for Rudolf Virchow, who first described its association with gastric cancer in 1848, refers to the metastatic involvement of the supraclavicular nodes at the junction of the thoracic duct and left subclavian vein.[3] In approximately 10% of patients with head and neck cancer, a clinically palpable metastatic lymph node is present without evidence of an obvious primary tumor. In these patients, a systematic workup is vital to establish an accurate tissue diagnosis in an effort to identify the occult primary tumor.

Patterns of neck metastasis

Metastases of cancer from primary sites in the upper aerodigestive tract to regional cervical lymph nodes usually occur in a foreseeable and sequential fashion. Many well-documented studies in the literature have shown that certain select groups of lymph nodes are initially at risk for dissemination to from each primary site in the head and neck region. Understanding the sequential pattern of metastasis is of importance when managing regions of at risk lymph nodes, lymph nodes at highest risk of harboring micrometastasis, especially in a clinically negative neck.

In primary tumors of the oral cavity, the regional cervical lymph nodes at highest risk of metastatic dissemination are levels I, II, and III.[4] When grouped together, levels I, II, and III are also known anatomically as the supraomohyoid triangle of the neck. Lymph node groups contained in these areas include the submental, submandibular, prevascular facial, superior spinal accessory, upper and mid jugular chains. Skip micrometastasis from the oral cavity to levels IV and V are less common. Thus, when the neck is clinically negative in level I to III, an elective neck dissection including levels IV and V are generally not necessary. An exception to this rule is that primary squamous cell carcinoma of the middle lateral third border of the tongue and floor of mouth have been shown to have skip metastases to level IV.[5] This fact has prompted some surgeons to abandon the supraomohyoid neck dissection in favor of a selective neck dissection, including levels I through IV for staging procedures of carcinomas of the lateral tongue.[6]

In primary tumors of the oropharynx, hypopharynx, and larynx, the regional cervical lymph nodes at highest risk for metastasis are levels II, III, and IV. The lymph node groups contained in these areas include the jugulodigastric, the superior spinal accessory, mid jugular, jugular-omohyoid, and supraclavicular lymph node chains. In primary tumors of the oropharynx, hypopharynx, and larynx, the risk of skip micrometastasis to levels I and V are rare without evidence of disease in levels II, III, or IV. Tumors in these areas that involve the midline are also at higher risk for metastatic dissemination to levels II, III, and IV on both sides of the neck. Of note, it has also been reported that tumors of the pyriform sinus have an increased risk of dissemination to the contralateral neck (Fig. 2).

The dissemination of metastasis from primary carcinomas of the parotid gland to regional lymph nodes has been reported to be in only 20% to 25% of the patients. The lymph node groups most at risk for dissemination are the preauricular, periparotid, and intraparotid chains surrounding the parotid gland as well as the upper deep jugular chain, level II, and upper spinal accessory chain in the posterior triangle of the neck, level V. In primary carcinomas of the submandibular salivary gland, the regional lymph node groups at highest risk are the submandibular, upper jugular, and mid jugular groups, also known as levels I, II, and III (Figs. 3 and 4).

The pattern of metastasis of cutaneous malignant tumors of the scalp, such as melanoma and cutaneous squamous cell carcinoma, is also predictable. An imaginary line is drawn in a coronal fashion joining the external auditory canal of one ear to that of the other ear. Primary tumors posterior to this line metastasize to the postauricular and suboccipital lymph node groups as well as the lymph nodes in the posterior triangle of the neck and the deep jugular chain (levels II–V). Primary tumors anterior to this line metastasize to the preauricular, preparotid, and anterior cervical lymph nodes (levels I–IV) with very rare metastasis to the posterior triangle of the neck.

Primary carcinomas of the thyroid gland also occur in a predictable pattern. The first level of lymph nodes at highest risk for metastasis is the perithyroid lymph nodes, which are adjacent to the thyroid gland, and those in the tracheoesophageal groove and superior mediastinum (levels V and VI) (Fig. 5). Metastatic disease from the thyroid gland carcinomas can progress sequentially from the lymph nodes in the tracheoesophageal groove to the lower deep jugular chain and then toward the mid and upper deep jugular chains and chains in the posterior triangle of the neck. Metastases from thyroid carcinomas to the submental and submandibular group of lymph nodes are very rare.

Metastatic neck disease staging

A uniform staging system of the cervical lymph nodes of head and neck cancer was put forth by the American Joint Committee on Cancer and the Union for International Cancer Control. It is the N portion of the TNM staging system (Table 1). The N staging system is reflective of the tumor burden of the lymph nodes and with the poorer prognosis with increasing N stage.[7]

History and physical examination

Neck masses have a higher risk of being malignant in older patients, especially those over the age of 40. During the history portion of the examination, a patient with tobacco or alcohol use, or both, with a neck mass present raises the suspicion of a malignant process. The duration of the mass is also important. Rapidly growing neck masses are commonly inflammatory; however, this can be seen with lymphomas. Patients who complain of dysphagia, dysphonia, and odynophagia are suspected of having primary oropharyngeal lesions. Fever, night sweats, unintended weight loss, the so-called "B" symptoms, are highly suggestive of lymphoma.

Physical examination findings differ depending on the malignancy with which the patient presents. Masses that are hard or fixed incite concern for malignancy. Often, these masses are tender. Cranial nerve palsies such as facial nerve weakness or accessory nerve weakness also suggest malignancy (Fig. 6).

A thorough head and neck examination should be performed to rule out cutaneous malignancies. A careful cranial nerve examination will identify ominous neural involvement and may assist in localization of the primary tumor. The thyroid gland should be palpated and any deviation of the trachea noted. The intraoral examination should include visualization of the oral mucosa and tongue but also bimanual palpation along the floor of the mouth and base of the tongue. In-office fiber optic nasopharyngoscopy is a simple, cost-effective adjunct to the direct physical examination. With topical anesthetic, most patients tolerate the procedure well. The nasal cavity, nasopharynx, oropharynx, and laryngeal inlet can all be visualized with the patient awake, and any abnormal function such as impaired vocal cord mobility or fixation of the epiglottis can be assessed.

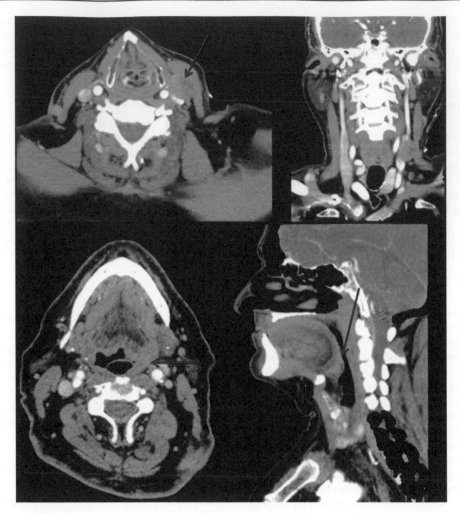

Fig. 2 CT from a 65-year-old man with a 50-pack-year smoking history. He presented with a complaint of a "lump" in his neck. Further questioning revealed intermittent dysphagia. No voice changes. Upper left image shows the axial contrast-enhanced lesion measuring 3 cm adjacent to the IJV and carotid artery, deep to the SCM (*red arrow*). Upper right image is a coronal rendering of the same lesion (*red arrow*). Lower left axial image shows asymmetry at the left base of tongue (*red arrow*). The lower right image is the left base of tongue lesion on sagittal rendering (*red arrow*). Biopsy demonstrated well-differentiated grade invasive squamous cell carcinoma.

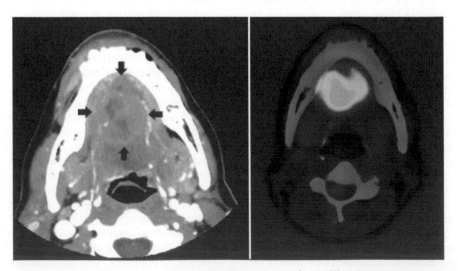

Fig. 3 CT and PET/CT from a 53-year-old woman with a right floor-of-mouth swelling (*black arrows*) of 4 months duration. She complained of dysphagia and dysphonia. She was a smoker and frequent alcohol user. Biopsy demonstrated high-grade mucoepidermoid carcinoma of the right submandibular salivary gland.

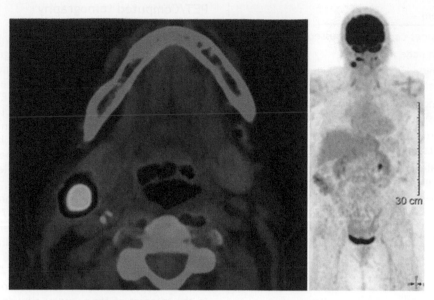

Fig. 4 PET/CT from a 74 year old woman with a complaint of a "lump" in her neck for a duration of 3 weeks. She did not complain of any pain. On physical examination, a matted, nontender mass in level II could be palpated. No cranial nerve deficits were noted. PET/CT shown demonstrates and FDG-avid mass in the tail of the parotid gland. Whole-body PET scan also demonstrates the lesion with no evidence of disease elsewhere. Patient was taken to the operating room for biopsy of the lesion. Frozen pathology suggested adenoid cystic carcinoma. A total parotidectomy was performed at that time.

Imaging

Anatomic, and increasingly functional, imaging is a critical adjunct in the workup of patients with neck masses. Many studies have been performed comparing the effectiveness and utility of the imaging modalities available. Each has certain strengths and limitations.

Computed tomography

Computed tomography (CT) imaging is a commonly used adjunct in the workup of the patients with head and neck cancer. CT imaging demonstrates superior spatial resolution and is best for evaluating bone invasion. Short acquisition times allow for less motion artifact and less exhausting experience for patients. CT is a useful adjunct to physical examination in staging tumors given the ability to identify invasion of deeper structures such as bone and vasculature. Although several characteristics of pathologically enlarged or distorted lymph nodes have been described in the literature, the sensitivity and specificity remain 83% for evaluating the neck for metastatic adenopathy.[8] Lymph nodes greater than 10 mm in diameter, the presence of central necrosis, rounded shape or loss of a normal fatty hilum, and increased or mixed uptake of

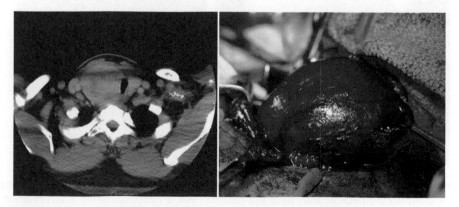

Fig. 5 A 41 year old man complaining of dysphagia with a central neck mass. Noncontrast CT demonstrating a 6-cm right thyroid mass extending into the supraclavicular space. Clinical photo showing extirpation of the well-circumscribed mass. Histologic evaluation revealed follicular thyroid carcinoma.

Table 1 N staging system

Nx	Regional lymph nodes cannot be assessed
N0	No regional lymph node metastasis
N1	Metastasis in a single ipsilateral lymph node, <3 cm in greatest dimension
N2a	Metastasis in a single ipsilateral lymph node, >3 cm in greatest dimension but <6 cm in greatest dimension
N2b	Metastases in multiple ipsilateral lymph nodes, none >6 cm in greatest dimension
N2c	Metastases in bilateral or contralateral lymph nodes, none >6 cm in greatest dimension
N3	Metastasis in a lymph node >6 cm in greatest dimension

Used with the permission of the American Joint Committee on Cancer (AJCC), Chicago, Illinois. The original source for this material is the AJCC Cancer Staging Manual, Seventh Edition (2010) published by Springer Science and Business Media LLC, http://www.springer.com.

contrast and obliteration of adjacent fat planes suggest carcinomatous involvement of the lymph node.

MRI

Although MRI produces superior definition of soft tissues as compared with CT, bony detail is inadequate. MRI is more effective in evaluating perineural spread, skull base invasion, and intracranial extension of head and neck cancer. With regards to evaluation of the neck, the sensitivity of MRI for detecting pathologic nodal metastases has been shown to be as low as 57%.[9]

PET/Computed tomography

PET with CT fusion imaging, also known as PET/CT, is becoming a commonly used tool in the oncologist's armamentarium for detection of, staging, and posttreatment surveillance of head and neck cancer. Although the National Comprehensive Cancer Network guidelines do not require PET/CT and the Radiation Therapy Oncology Group does not include PET/CT as a staging tool, many oncologists and cancer centers are using PET/CT in the management of patients with head and neck cancer. Several limitations of PET/CT must be kept in mind. This modality lacks the sensitivity to detect lesions less than 5 mm in the smallest dimension. In addition, this modality does not differentiate malignancy versus inflammation or tissues with high baseline metabolic activity (Fig. 7). Therefore, caution for overzealous treatment should be exercised. Accordingly, it is generally not recommended to obtain surveillance posttreatment PET/CT imaging sooner than 8 weeks after treatment because of residual inflammation.[10] Also, many patients present for biopsy of an oral lesion before obtaining any imaging. In the interest of time, many clinicians will proceed with biopsy and then obtain the scan. Inflammation due to the biopsy may lead to false positive results on PET/CT imaging. The sensitivity and specificity for PET/CT imaging has been shown to be 98 and 93% with a positive predictive value of 63% and a negative predictive value of 99.7%.[11]

Fine needle aspiration biopsy

The use of ultrasound (US) -guided fine-needle aspiration biopsy (FNAB) in the evaluation of patients with head and neck cancer has been demonstrated to be safe, and under US guidance, has similar sensitivity and specificity to contrast CT in identifying pathologically enlarged lymph nodes.[8,12] In addition, CT and US-guided FNA have similar overall accuracy

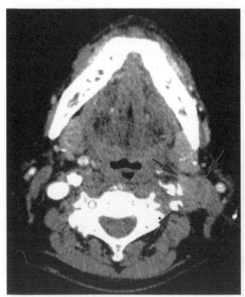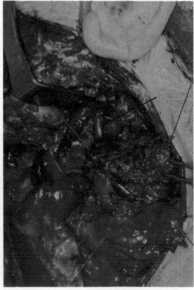

Fig. 6 An 87 year old woman with a history of a 1.8-cm squamous cell carcinoma of the left retromolar trigone removed 3 years before presentation. Patient had a clinically N0 neck at that time and refused neck dissection. During a surveillance visit, a neck mass was palpated in the left level II area. On further questioning, she had difficulty raising her arm to apply deodorant. CT showing a 1.8-cm mass with compression of the IJV and loss of normal fat planes around the SCM (*thick red arrows*). Clinical photograph demonstrating the mass (*thin red arrows*) directly involving the spinal accessory nerve (*thin black arrow*).

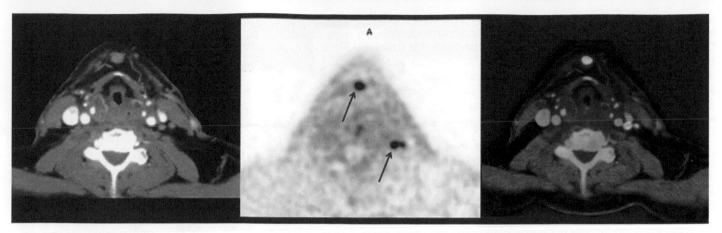

Fig. 7 Routine surveillance PET/CT from a 74-year-old man with a history of T1 supraglottic laryngeal squamous cell carcinoma treated with chemotherapy and radiation therapy 4 years prior and a second primary T1 floor-of-mouth squamous cell carcinoma treated with wide local excision 2 years prior. Note the FDG avid nodes in levels I and II of the left neck (*red arrows*, center, corresponding contrast CT to the left, and PET/CT to the right). Patient underwent neck dissection. Pathology results were negative for malignancy.

in terms of sampling neck lymph nodes and are both superior to palpation alone.[13] The value of performing US-guided FNAB is that it is an oncologically safe procedure with little morbidity that can be performed under local anesthesia in the surgeon's office. An experienced cytologist can give preliminary results within a matter of minutes. Caution in interpreting negative results is warranted. Negative FNAB should either be repeated or an oncologically appropriate open biopsy be performed.

Management of the neck

G.W. Crile, in 1906, was first credited with describing the first "radical neck dissection," and several other authors have proposed modifications since.[14] More recently, in 2008, the American Head and Neck Society committee on neck dissections developed a standard approach to the description of the neck dissection, which is based on a modification of the radical neck dissection (Table 2).

Prescribing the proper neck dissection

Choice of neck dissection is based on the patient's preoperative clinical examination and stage of disease. Advanced tumors with known or suspected extensive lymph node metastasis or involvement of the spinal accessory nerve or IJV should undergo a radical neck dissection. Similarly, a modified

radical neck dissection should be considered when the patient presents with grossly visible lymph node disease that is not suspected to directly infiltrate nonlymphatic structures. Nerve palsy, restriction in range of motion, or preoperative imaging demonstrating loss of usual fat planes between structures or compression of the IJV should make the surgeon suspicious. Often, the decision to perform a radical neck dissection versus a modified radical neck dissection is made intraoperatively.

Many authors consider the selective neck dissection a staging procedure. Tumors of the oral cavity, pharynx, and hypopharynx in which the risk of subclinical nodal disease (ie, "occult" metastasis) is greater than 15%, and there is no indication for a radical or modified radical neck dissection, a selective neck dissection is often prescribed to rule out the presence of metastatic disease. Selective neck dissection is useful in determining whether the patient will require adjuvant chemotherapy, radiation therapy, or both as well as accurate staging and prognostication.

Procedure for performing a neck dissection

Although a thorough description of the various techniques and nuances of performing a neck dissection is out of the scope of this article, a brief description follows.

First, a utility incision is marked. Landmarks include the mastoid process, inferior border of the mandible, the clavicle,

Table 2	American Head and Neck Society neck dissection classification
Radical neck dissection	Removal of lymphatic tissues in levels I–V along with the SCM, IJV, and spinal accessory nerve (SAN)
Modified radical neck dissection	Removal of lymphatic tissues in levels I–V with preservation of one or more nonlymphatic structures: Type III: preservation of SCM, IJV, SAN Type II: preservation of IJV, SAN Type I: preservation of SAN
Extended neck dissection	Removal of additional lymphatic tissue and/or nonlymphatic structures not normally removed in a radical neck dissection
Selective neck dissection	Preservation of one or more lymphatic levels as well as nonlymphatic structures normally removed in a radical neck dissection

Adapted from Robbins KT, Shaha AR, Medina JE, et al. Consensus statement on the classification and terminology of neck dissection. Arch Otolaryngol Head Neck Surg 2008;134(5):536–8.

and midline chin. The incision is centered in a skin crease between the inferior border of the mandible and the clavicle. Often, the external jugular vein is marked because this structure is preserved for lateral microvascular anastomosis and it commonly serves as a landmark for locating the greater auricular nerve, which usually lies in the same plane within 1 cm posterior to the external jugular vein (Fig. 8). Once the incision is marked, the skin is infiltrated with epinephrine-containing local anesthetic.

Next, the skin incision is made and carried through the platysma. Subplatysmal flaps are elevated to the level of the inferior border of the mandible superiorly and the clavicle inferiorly. Care is taken to avoid leaving any fibrolymphatic tissue attached to the platysma. If the neck dissection is performed concurrently with a tracheotomy, care is also taken to prevent communication of the inferior skin-platysmal flap with the tracheotomy wound. Once the flaps are elevated, they are retracted with stay sutures or hooks.

For a radical neck dissection or modified radical neck dissection with sacrifice of the (SCM, the SCM is freed from its attachments to the mastoid and clavicle. Then, level V lymph nodes are dissected and the spinal accessory nerve is preserved if possible. Level V lymph nodes along with the SCM, level II, III, and IV lymph nodes are dissected in an anterior direction. During dissection of levels III and IV, care is taken to avoid injury to the lymphatic ducts, phrenic nerve, vagus nerve, or brachial plexus (Fig. 9). If the IJV is to be sacrificed, it is ligated proximally and distally and then dissected in continuity with the specimen. If the IJV is to be left in place, careful removal of the fascia and lymphatic tissue circumferentially around the IJV is performed while avoiding excessive torsion on the vein. Branches emanating from the vein on the anterior and medial surface are ligated and divided. The entire specimen is dissected further off of the carotid artery, taking care not to excessively thin the carotid artery or injure the vagus nerve. Next, level I lymph nodes are dissected starting in level IA and moving posterior. The facial nerve is identified and dissected free of the fascia and retracted superiorly; this allows complete dissection of level IB and the perifacial lymph nodes while protecting the facial nerve from inadvertent injury.

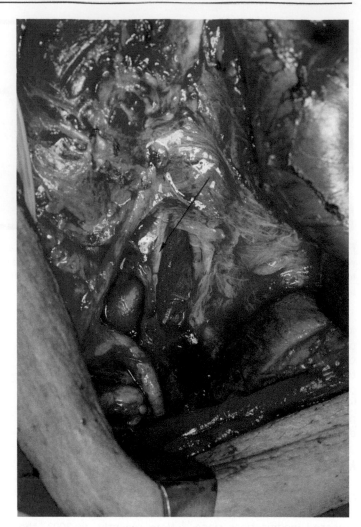

Fig. 9 Dissection of level IV. Note the phrenic nerve (*black arrow*). The IJV is retracted medially and the sternocleidomastoid is dissected laterally.

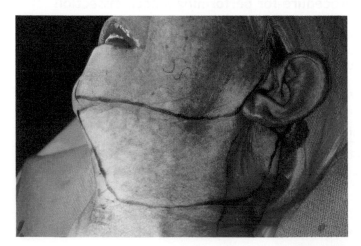

Fig. 8 Typical utility incision useful for most neck dissections. Vertical line marking the external jugular vein. An incision placed posteriorly over the sternocleidomastoid can be placed for added exposure of the clavicle, level IV, and the attachments of the sternocleidomastoid. Care must be taken to avoid placing a trifurcation suture line over the carotid artery.

The mylohyoid muscle is identified and retracted anteriorly, and the submandibular duct, lingual nerve, and hypoglossal nerves are identified. The duct is ligated and divided, and the gland along with the nodal contents of the submandibular triangle is then delivered inferiorly. By this point, the specimen is held only by some attachments immediately anterior to the carotid artery. These attachments are carefully divided taking care not to injure branches of the external carotid artery. Once this is complete, the specimen is delivered from the neck. Fig. 10 shows a completed radical neck dissection with removal of nodes in levels I through V along with removal of the SCM, IJV, and spinal accessory nerve.

A selective neck dissection proceeds in the same manner as a modified radical neck dissection or radical neck dissection with several changes to facilitate preservation of nonlymphatic structures. In a selective neck dissection, once the subplatysmal flaps are elevated, the fascia over the SCM is incised and the SCM is retracted laterally to expose level II, III, and IV lymph nodes. These levels are then dissected from the fascia over the splenius capitus and levator scapulae muscles, taking care not to injure the spinal accessory nerve, phrenic nerve, brachial plexus, or lymphatic ducts. The specimen is brought anterior as the dissection proceeds. Dissection of the IJV proceeds with care not to injure the vein, the vagus nerve, or

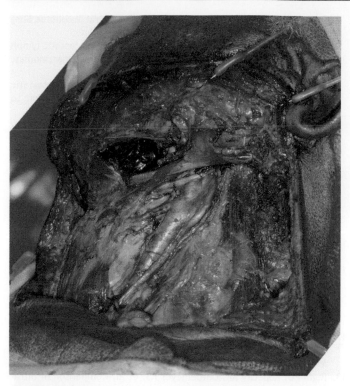

Fig. 10 Completed radical neck dissection. Note the removal of the sternocleidomastoid, the IJV, and spinal accessory nerve along with nodes levels I–V.

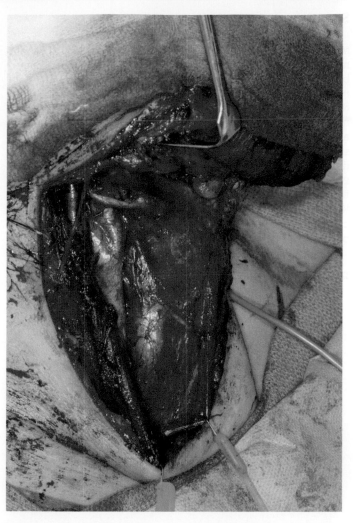

Fig. 11 Completed selective neck dissection. Note preservation of the great auricular nerve, SCM, and IJV. Not shown is the intact spinal accessory nerve, which is preserved in a selective neck dissection.

carotid artery. Dissection of level I proceeds in the same manner as for a modified radical or radical neck dissection. Fig. 11 shows a completed selective neck dissection with an intact great auricular nerve, an intact SCM, and an intact IJV. Once the specimen is removed, it is oriented for the pathologist and the levels are marked with skin staples or sutures (Fig. 12). Drains are placed in the wound and the wound is closed, reapproximating platysma with Vicryl suture and skin with staples.

Pearls and pitfalls in performing neck dissection

When designing the skin incision, care must be taken to avoid trifurcation incisions over carotid artery because postoperative skin breakdown (often secondary to soft tissue radiation injury) can lead to carotid exposure and blowout. If additional access is required for removal of the SCM, a vertical incision connecting to the utility incision is placed as far posterior as possible. In a selective neck dissection during dissection of levels II and III, the surgeon should use the posterior border of the SCM as a landmark to avoid dissecting level V. The dissection should be carried in a medial direction. When dissecting level II, the surgeon should keep in mind the proximity of the IJV to the spinal accessory nerve to avoid injury and a troublesome bleed. When dissecting level IIA and IB, it is useful to keep in mind that the area superficial to the posterior belly of the digastric muscle is safe, and this area can be dissected relatively quickly. When dissecting level III, there is a thin fascia at the level of the transverse cervical nerves and, although the transverse cervical nerves can be sacrificed in most people without detriment, others derive a significant

amount of trapezius innervations by the transverse cervical nerves. Leaving the transverse cervical nerves in place and dissecting lymphatic tissue anterior to these nerves allows the surgeon to more easily define the plane of dissection.

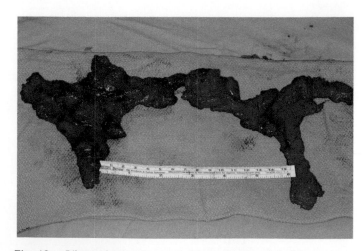

Fig. 12 Bilateral selective neck dissection (levels I–IV) specimen taken en bloc from the neck.

Summary

Metastatic neck masses can represent a variety of local or distant malignant diseases. The differential diagnosis can be tailored based on a thorough history and physical examination and an understanding of patient risk factors and patterns of metastasis. New neck masses in the adult patient should be considered malignant until proven otherwise. There are several diagnostic adjuncts in the workup of the neck mass and each has its strengths and weaknesses. If used within the confines of their limitations, these tests can result in a timely, accurate, and cost-effective workup. Of utmost importance is accurate diagnosis of the source of the metastatic neck disease. Management of malignant neck mass itself often consists of surgical treatment, although radiation and/or chemotherapy may also be appropriate depending on the clinical scenario.

References

1. Haksever M, Inançlı HM, Tunçel U, et al. The effects of tumor size, degree of differentiation, and depth of invasion on the risk of neck node metastasis in squamous cell carcinoma of the oral cavity. Ear Nose Throat J 2012;91(3):130—5.
2. Thompson C, St John M, Lawson G, et al. Diagnostic value of sentinel lymph node biopsy in head and neck cancer: a meta-analysis. Eur Arch Otorhinolaryngol 2013;270(7):2115—22.
3. Siosaki MD, Souza AT. Images in clinical medicine. Virchow's node. N Engl J Med 2013;368:e7.
4. Woolgar JA. The topography of cervical lymph node metastases revisited: the histological findings in 526 sides of neck dissection from 439 previously untreated patients. Int J Oral Maxillofac Surg 2007;36(3):219—25.
5. Tao L, Lefèvre M, Callard P, et al. Reappraisal of metastatic lymph node topography in head and neck squamous cell carcinomas. Otolaryngol Head Neck Surg 2006;135(3):445—50.
6. Crean SJ, Hoffman A, Potts J, et al. Reduction of occult metastatic disease by extension of the supraomohyoid neck dissection to include level IV. Head Neck 2003;25(9):758—62.
7. Edge SB, Byrd DR, Compton CC, et al, editors. AJCC cancer staging manual. 7th edition. New York: Springer; 2010.
8. Robitschek J, Straub M, Wirtz E, et al. Diagnostic efficacy of surgeon-performed ultrasound-guided fine needle aspiration: a randomized controlled trial. Otolaryngol Head Neck Surg 2010; 142(3):306—9.
9. Lee J, Fernandes R. Neck masses: evaluation and diagnostic approach. Oral Maxillofac Surg Clin North Am 2008;20(3): 321—37.
10. Johnson JT, Branstetter BF 4th. PET/CT in head and neck oncology: State-of-the-art 2013. Laryngoscope 2014;124(4):913—5.
11. Kim SY, Roh JL, Yeo NK, et al. Combined 18F-fluorodeoxyglucose-positron emission tomography and computed tomography as a primary screening method for detecting second primary cancers and distant metastases in patients with head and neck cancer. Ann Oncol 2007;18(10):1698.
12. Saatian M, Badie BM, Shahriari S, et al. FNA diagnostic value in patients with neck masses in two teaching hospitals in Iran. Acta Med Iran 2011;49(2):85—8.
13. Righi PD, Kopecky KK, Caldemeyer KS, et al. Comparison of ultrasound-fine needle aspiration and computed tomography in patients undergoing elective neck dissection. Head Neck 1997;19(7):604.
14. Subramanian S, Chiesa F, Lyubaev V, et al. The evolution of surgery in the management of neck metastasis. Acta Otorhinolaryngol Ital 2006;26(6):309—16.

Reconstruction of Cervical Defects

Tuan G. Bui, MD, DMD [a,b,]*, Eric J. Dierks, MD, DMD [a,b]

KEYWORDS

- Cervical defect • Larynx • Hypopharynx • Reconstruction • Esophagus

KEY POINTS

- Reconstruction of various cervical defects can be quite challenging; prior oncologic resection combined with radiation therapy compounds the level of difficulty.
- The judicious application of vascularized flaps, either pedicled or free flaps, can significantly improve the quality of life of cancer survivors with these issues.
- To prevent or reduce the incidence of postoperative pharyngocutaneous fistulas or esophageal strictures, a variety of pedicled or free flaps can be used. Some surgeons temporary use a salivary bypass tube to potentially further decrease the risk of pharyngocutaneous fistulas.

Introduction

The topic of reconstruction of cervical defects can entail a wide range of patient problems and possible solutions. This article is limited to the anterior and lateral neck region, where the level of complexity of the reconstruction of defects can be compounded by the prior use of ionizing radiation. Although most reconstructions are related to oncologic defects and the complications arising from such treatment, these techniques can be equally applicable to traumatic and other causes. Specific topics covered include pharyngeal and cervical esophageal reconstruction, pharyngocutaneous fistula (PCF) repair, carotid artery coverage, release of cervical wound contracture, and correction of esophageal stricture and cutaneous cervical defects.

Pharyngeal and cervical esophageal reconstruction

Patients with tumors involving the larynx or hypopharynx can be a reconstructive challenge. After completion of the ablative surgery, part of the reconstructive task is to repair or recreate a conduit from the base of tongue to the proximal cervical esophagus. In the nonirradiated neck that has not previously been operated on, this can usually be accomplished with good success via primary closure of the residual pharyngeal mucosa. The minimum amount of mucosa this requires is approximately 2.5 cm.[1]

To prevent or reduce the incidence of postoperative PCFs or esophageal strictures, a variety of pedicled or free flaps can be used. Some surgeons temporarily use a salivary bypass tube to potentially further decrease the risk of PCFs.

Pectoralis major myocutaneous flap

The pectoralis major myocutaneous (PMMC) flap, originally described by Ariyan,[2] is a reliable and robust flap that provides extensive well-vascularized tissue; one of its potential drawbacks can be the excessive amount of tissue. Furthermore, it is an easy flap to harvest, and does not require microvascular skills, thereby decreasing operative time.

The skin portion of the flap can be used to reconstruct the pharynx by suturing the edges to the residual mucosal edges, or by tubing it in cases of circumferential pharyngeal defects. The muscle adds a second layer of vascularized tissue between the pharyngeal closure and cervical skin, which decreases the risk of PCF. The muscle can also be used to cover and protect the carotid artery in irradiated patients. A skin graft can be used to cover the area of exposed muscle if the clinician is unable to primarily close the cervical skin.

The rate of PCF formation with the use of PMMC flap has been reported to be approximately 10% to 15%, compared with 36% to 50% without the flap.[3,4] Studies have shown a median esophageal stenosis rate of approximately 17% with the use of a PMMC flap,[5] versus 33% without it.[6]

Drawbacks of the PMMC flap for pharyngeal reconstruction can include impaired swallowing and speech articulation if a significant portion of the base of tongue is involved. The weight of the flap can pull the residual tongue down, causing difficulty with speech and swallowing. This effect can be minimized by suturing the flap down to the prevertebral fascia. Other drawbacks include limitation of contralateral neck turning, and a bulky area where the flap traverses over the clavicle, although this may improve with time with muscle atrophy. Furthermore, patients can experience postoperative shoulder joint dysmotility.

[a] Oral and Maxillofacial Surgery, Oregon Health and Sciences University, Portland, OR, USA
[b] Head and Neck Surgical Institute, 1849 Northwest Kearney Street, #300, Portland, OR 97209, USA
* Corresponding author. Head and Neck Surgical Institute, 1849 Northwest Kearney Street, #300, Portland, OR 97209.
E-mail address: tgbui@hnsa1.com

Atlas Oral Maxillofacial Surg Clin N Am 23 (2015) 105–115
1061-3315/15/$ - see front matter © 2015 Elsevier Inc. All rights reserved.
http://dx.doi.org/10.1016/j.cxom.2014.10.006

Supraclavicular artery island flap

The anatomy of the supraclavicular artery island flap (SCAIF) was originally described by Toldt.[7] This flap is based off the supraclavicular artery, which typically branches from the thyrocervical trunk. It is easy to harvest, with minimal donor site morbidity. It provides thin and pliable tissue; ideal for head and neck reconstruction. For pharyngeal defects, it can be used as a patch graft or as a tubed, interpositional graft. The rate of PCF with the use of SCAIF has been reported to be approximately 20%.[8]

Fasciocutaneous free flaps

Multiple fasciocutaneous free flaps have been described for use in the head and neck region. However, the radial forearm free flap (RFFF) and anterolateral thigh (ALT) free flap, described by Yang and colleagues[9] and Song and colleagues,[10] are the most widely used flaps for soft tissue reconstruction in the head and neck region.

Their use in the reconstruction of pharyngeal and cervical esophageal defects is well recognized. Their ease of harvest, even with the anatomic variation associated with the ALT, and minimal donor site morbidity, make them attractive options. The vessel diameter of both vascular pedicles is large, allowing easier vascular anastomoses, which is particularly important in previously irradiated necks. Although the ALT flap allows a larger amount of tissue to be harvested, both flaps can be designed and used in multiple ways to adequately reconstruct the defect. However, inherent in the use of microvascular free flaps is the risk of flap failure, which, although low, can have serious consequences. The increase in operating time may also be detrimental to patients, particularly for those who are medically compromised, as are most patients with head and neck defects (Figs. 1–5).

The mean rates of PCF and esophageal stenosis for the RFFF and ALT flaps are less than 25% and around 10%, respectively.[5] It has also been reported that patients who have been reconstructed using either of these fasciocutaneous free flaps have perhaps the best recovery in terms of voice rehabilitation and swallowing function compared with all other forms of reconstruction (Figs. 6–8).[5,11]

Jejunal free flaps

The jejunal free flap was originally described by Seidenberg and colleagues,[12] and is the oldest form of circumferential pharyngeal reconstruction still being used. Patients who have received this form of reconstruction typically have good voice rehabilitation and swallowing capabilities. The PCF and stricture rates are similar to those of the fasciocutaneous free flaps. However, their decreased operative ischemia time and high morbidity rate, compared with the fasciocutaneous free flaps, have led to their decreased use.[5]

Pharyngocutaneous fistula repair

The neck can be the site of a variety of PCFs, often arising following laryngectomy or laryngopharyngectomy, particularly in previously irradiated patients. Many PCFs following laryngectomy are successfully managed by standard measures, such as the use of a nasogastric or gastrostomy feeding tubes, keeping the patient nil by mouth optimization of thyroid function, and serial wound packing, thus allowing them to heal

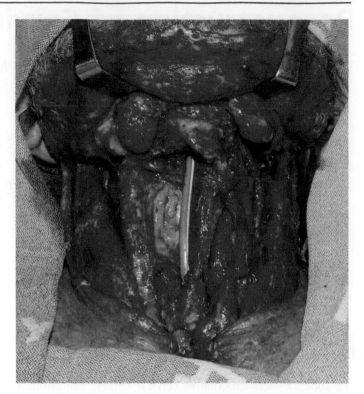

Fig. 1 Defect after total laryngectomy and partial pharyngectomy in a previously irradiated patient. There is a remnant of posterior hypopharynx present. The nasogastric tube passes into the cervical esophagus.

by secondary intention. Therefore, most PCFs should be managed conservatively for an extended period of time, with surgical intervention and reconstruction reserved only for defects that have proved refractory to local measures and nutritional optimization.

For persistent PCF, surgical intervention is required, which entails resection of the fistula, and flaps to reconstruct the residual defect. Similar to the partial pharyngeal defect repair described earlier, flaps commonly used for persistent PCF are the PMMC, SCAIF, and RFFF, either alone or in combination. A skin graft may also be required if primary closure of the cervical skin is not possible (Figs. 9 and 10).

Smaller fistulae occurring in the region of a tracheal stoma in the lower neck can occasionally be addressed using a local sternocleidomastoid flap rotated medially. This procedure should not be attempted in previously irradiated patients. A

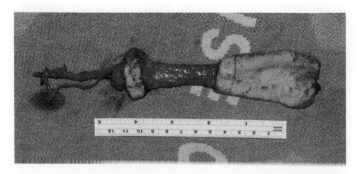

Fig. 2 Harvested RFFF with separate skin paddle for external monitoring.

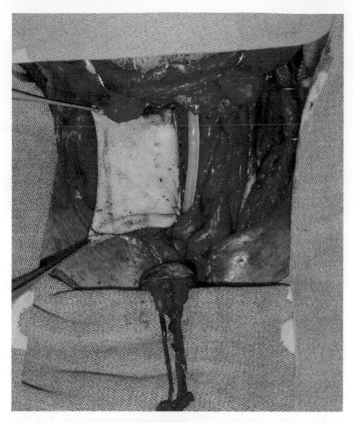

Fig. 3 Partial inset of the RFFF. The skin edges of the flap are sutured to the edges of the remaining hypopharyngeal mucosa, base of tongue, and cervical esophagus.

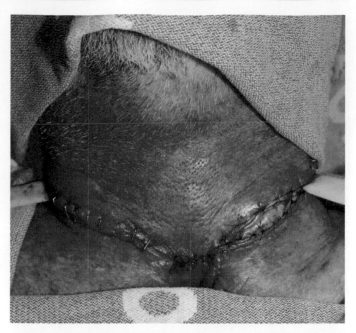

Fig. 5 Closure of cervical wound with external skin paddle from RFFF for flap monitoring.

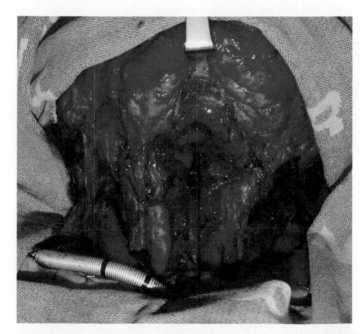

Fig. 6 Defect after total laryngectomy and total pharyngectomy. Note that there is no remaining hypopharyngeal mucosa.

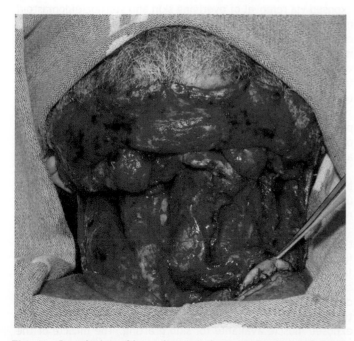

Fig. 4 Completion of hypopharyngeal reconstruction with RFFF.

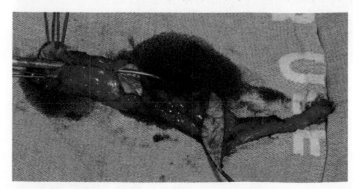

Fig. 7 Harvested RFFF that has been tubed for eventual replacement of the hypopharynx.

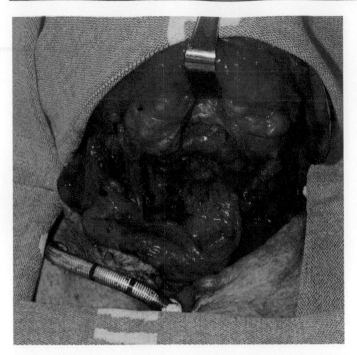

Fig. 8   The tubed RFFF has been inset and sutured to the base of tongue and cervical esophagus to replace the hypopharynx.

more reliable source of vascularized and nonirradiated tissue is the pedicled pectoralis major myocutaneous or myofascial flap.

Carotid artery coverage

The carotid artery can be exposed in a variety of settings, almost all of which are related to surgery and/or radiation therapy for head and neck cancer. The most frequent such

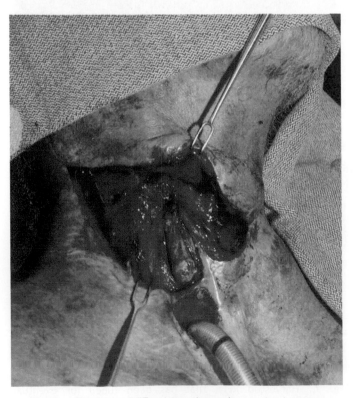

Fig. 9   Persistent PCF exiting above the tracheal stoma.

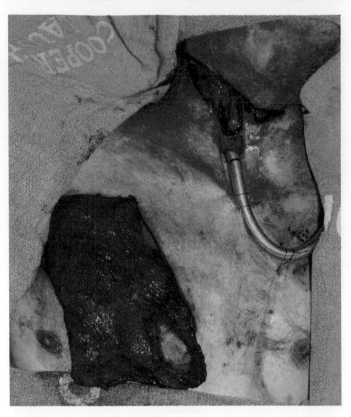

Fig. 10   Harvested pectoralis major myocutaneous flap. The flap is tunneled under the bridging skin to reach the fistula. The skin paddle from the flap is used to reconstruct the pharyngeal defect, and a skin graft is placed over the exposed pectoralis muscle to complete the closure of the cervical skin.

situation involves salvage surgery in which a patient who has undergone prior resection and a full course of radiotherapy then undergoes reoperation in an attempt to remove recurrent tumor. Because such surgeries are typically, at a minimum, radical neck dissections, and more frequently are extended radical neck dissections, the carotid artery may either be exposed via removal of overlying skin and sternocleidomastoid muscle or may be resected and replaced with a vascular conduit graft. In either situation, a vascularized reconstruction is necessary to ensure the viability of the reconstruction. The vascularized flap should provide an insulating, enveloping bed for the carotid artery, or the carotid reconstruction extending to, and usually replacing, the overlying skin. On the deep side, such radical resections frequently enter into the nearby pharynx, and the reconstruction must also provide a water-proof barrier to prohibit saliva from contaminating the carotid and its reconstruction.

To make matters even more challenging, the neck in these patients is often severely vessel depleted; therefore, we often use pedicled flaps in these instances, because of their high reliability.

The PMMC is a reliable, bulky, and well-vascularized flap that is ideal to reconstruct such defects. The pectoralis major flap can be extended to and above the level of the angle of the jaw and can carry a viable skin paddle for cover (external coverage) or lining (internal reconstruction of a mucosal defect). Here, an elliptically shaped skin paddle may be used to reconstruct the mucosal defect, leaving the external exposed muscle available for skin grafting. The muscle of the pectoralis major flap, as well as a thin skin paddle, can also be

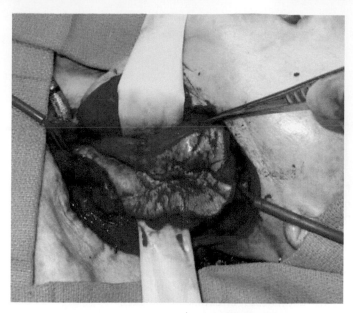

Fig. 11 Recurrent cancer involving the left common carotid artery, internal jugular vein, sternocleidomastoid, and overlying skin.

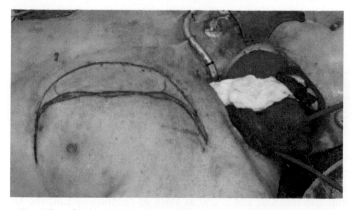

Fig. 12 Outline of the pectoralis major myocutaneous flap.

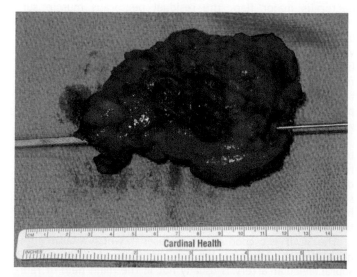

Fig. 13 Resected specimen including the common carotid and internal carotid arteries.

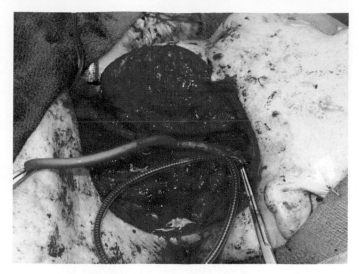

Fig. 14 A vascular shunt was used during the repair of the common carotid—internal carotid artery system.

used as an internal reconstruction for missing lateral pharyngeal wall (Figs. 11—16).

Postoperative wound healing problems are common in this scenario. Although the transposed pectoralis muscle flap has a robust blood supply, clinicians must keep in mind that the recipient tissue bed has been radiated and may be slow to integrate with the reconstructive flap. For this reason, surgeons must ensure that suspensory sutures are placed throughout the wound field, anchoring the flap to prevertebral or other adjacent fascial structures. Prolonged passive drainage of the prevertebral area can be helpful in avoiding fluid collections and failure.

Larger neck defects are best managed via a pedicled latissimus dorsi myocutaneous flap, tunneled through the axilla.

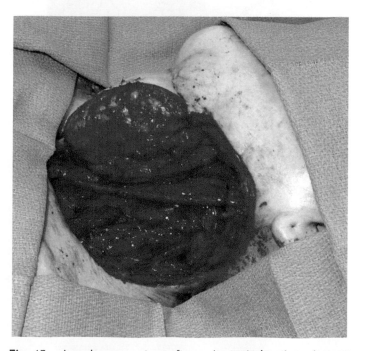

Fig. 15 A saphenous vein graft was harvested and used as an interpositional vascular graft to reconstruct the common carotid—internal carotid artery system.

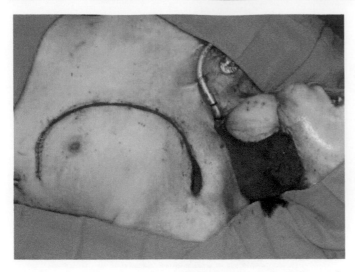

Fig. 16 Rotation of the PMMC flap into the neck to cover the reconstructed common carotid—internal carotid artery system. A skin graft is placed over the exposed pectoralis muscle. Primary closure of the chest wound.

The latissimus dorsi flap is reliable, although care must be taken to avoid kinking of the venous outflow when rotating it into the neck. Increasing the arc of rotation of the flap can be achieved by releasing the muscle attachment to the humerus, which can also be done for the PMMC. An additional technical note for when a PMMC or latissimus dorsi flap is harvested for use in this setting is that it can be helpful to use the GIA stapler to divide the muscles from their insertions. The row of ministaples makes the muscle easier to securely suture into place (Figs. 17—20).

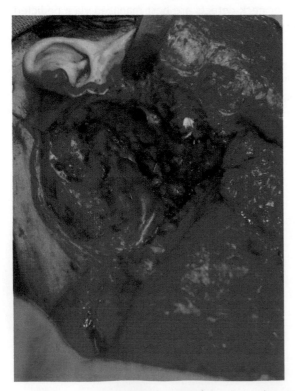

Fig. 17 Defect showing exposed internal jugular vein, carotid arteries, lateral pharyngeal defect, and extending up to the skull base in a previously irradiated patient.

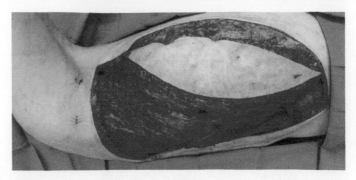

Fig. 18 Harvested pedicled latissimus dorsi muscle myocutaneous flap. A large skin paddle ensures capture of the skin perforators.

The chimeric vastus lateralis—ALT flap is a good free flap option.[13] This flap contains an abundance of tissue that can be used to protect the carotid artery, fill in dead space, and reconstruct mucosal or cutaneous defects.

Release of cervical wound contracture

Neck reconstruction for cervical wound contracture can offer a significant improvement in quality of life for cancer survivors who experience scar contracture with resultant limitation of cervical range of motion. The combination of surgery and radiation therapy provides a potent stimulus for scar contracture, which can occur years after successful cancer treatment. Contractures frequently occur along the ridge of the anterior border of the sternocleidomastoid muscle, even if the muscle has been removed. Contractures and scar banding in this area can also involve the pedicle of a previously placed pectoralis major muscle.

The judicious use of large Z-plasties can greatly improve the situation, release the scar, and often improve the rotational range of motion of the head and neck. The Z-plasty should be of a standard 60° design and should be performed in such a way that the limbs of the Z are as thick as reasonably possible to ensure viability of the overlying skin. Once the arms of the Z have been elevated, regional undermining allows transposition. If the Z-plasty is performed over the pedicle of a pectoralis major flap, the residual pectoralis muscle surrounding the pedicle should be excised, preserving the thoracoacromial artery and adjacent vein to ensure continued viability of the previously placed flap. Transposition of the limbs of the Z-plasty may be accompanied by some tension and further release may be needed. It is incumbent on the surgeon to preserve flap thickness to ensure viability of the subdermal plexus. Following transposition, the flaps are sutured in place with buried resorbable suture and skin staples.

In irradiated patients it is common for the repaired wounds to undergo a period of wound breakdown. This breakdown requires local wound care, and potentially even partial debridement of the wound edges. Nonetheless, healing does slowly progress and, once the wound dehiscence has slowly healed by secondary intention, the benefit of the Z-plasty transposition is realized (Figs. 21—24).

The SCAIF is a good option in cases in which a large cutaneous defect arises after the scar contracture is released. The supraclavicular artery is usually not in the main field of radiation, and is typically not dissected out during surgery, thereby making this flap highly reliable for use in this situation.

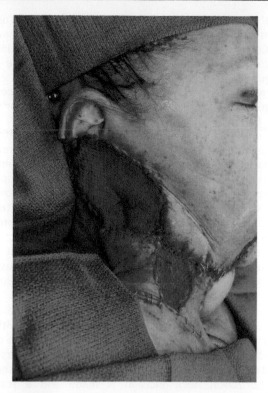

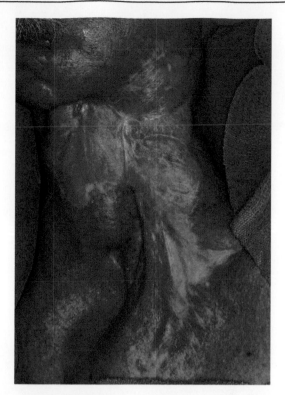

Fig. 19 Final inset of the latissimus dorsi muscle flap. The skin paddle was used to reconstruct the lateral pharyngeal defect. The large amount of available muscle was used to cover the neck vessels, line the skull base, and fill in the dead space. Skin grafts were used to cover the exposed muscle.

Fig. 21 Cervical scar contracture from a previous PMMC flap in an irradiated patient. Note the tight scar band that formed along the path of the rotated pectoralis muscle.

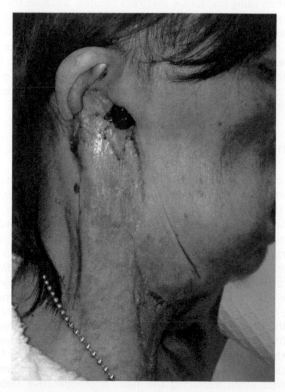

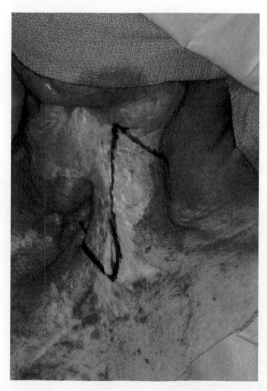

Fig. 20 Healing of the flap and wound. Note the presence of the cervical scar contracture, which is common with the use of local, pedicled flaps.

Fig. 22 Design of the Z-plasty, with the long axis of the Z along the length of the scar.

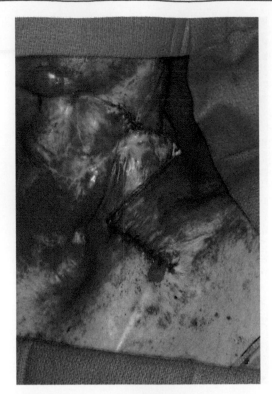

Fig. 23 Completion of the Z-plasty, with release of the cervical scar contracture.

Correction of cervical esophageal stricture

In patients having laryngectomy or laryngopharyngectomy, primary defect closure without the interposition of a microvascular free flap can result in circumferential stenosis. Radiation therapy is virtually always a major component of these

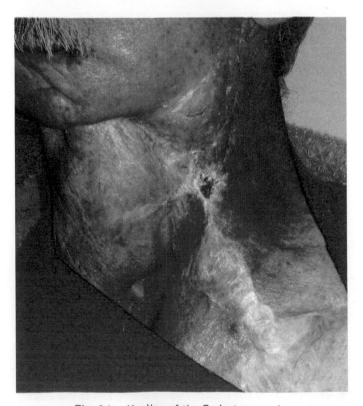

Fig. 24 Healing of the Z-plasty wounds.

patients' oncologic management and the stenotic site is usually centered within the maximum dosage area, which may exceed 70 Gy. Complete stenosis requires an endoscopic rendezvous procedure to connect the cervical esophagus with the distal esophagus. These esophagi often restenose, and total esophagectomy with gastric pull-up reconstruction or cervical esophagectomy with reconstruction with a tubed ALT or radial forearm flap may be required.

More commonly, the cervical esophagus remains patent at the site of stenosis, but the focal, hourglass narrowing remains problematic. This narrowing produces a significant diminution of quality of life of patients after laryngectomy and can also adversely affect esophageal speech. A barium swallow can identify the site of the stenosis, which can be dilated via endoscopic balloon dilation. Serial bougie dilation can produce transient improvement in this type of stenosis but the stenotic area usually reforms. Some patients become adept at home dilation and can maintain their dilation with the home use of a bougie, but others are not successful and require open surgical repair.

An inlay of a thin and pliable fasciocutaneous flap is an ideal reconstruction for the stenotic sites. This flap can be either in the form of a pedicled SCAIF or an RFFF. The operation begins with placement of a bougie from the mouth into the esophagus to facilitate identification of the esophagus during dissection. A low horizontal neck incision is made and a standard dissection is performed over the tracheal stoma. The tracheaesophageal groove is opened without entry into the membranous posterior wall of the trachea. The underlying esophagus is circumferentially dissected. The site of the stenosis is usually easy to identify. A vertical incision is made through this stenosis and is extended both proximally and distally to allow insertion of an oval-shaped inlay. The fasciocutaneous flap is trimmed to fit the defect and is inserted with the skin side into the lumen using horizontal mattress sutures. Because the flap will not be accessible for direct monitoring, the use of an external skin paddle is optional. A nasogastric tube is placed unless the patient already has a gastrostomy tube. Because of the inevitable salivary leakage around the flap inlay site, consideration should be given to leaving passive drains in place for 7 to 10 days. We advise waiting at least 2 weeks before resuming oral intake (Figs. 25–30).

Cutaneous cervical defects

Large cutaneous defects of the neck can be created in situations in which deeper tissues are uninvolved. Such problems arise from the excision of cutaneous malignancies or the excision of poorly healed scar tissue that cannot be closed via Z-plasty or other local tissue rearrangement. The cervicalpectoral rotation-advancement flap (CPF) is reliable and can be used in these situations. It offers the advantage of similar skin color and texture, but may require a second stage to reduce a standing cone at the site of rotation. The CPF should not be considered if the patient has had a previous transverse neck incision, or if the patient has had a previous deltopectoral flap. The CPF draws its vascular supply from perforators from the mammary artery. Perforators numbers 2 and 4 are classically described, and all available perforators should be preserved when elevating the flap. A preoperative Doppler examination of the neck may help to identify and mark the sites of the perforators along the lateral border of the sternum.

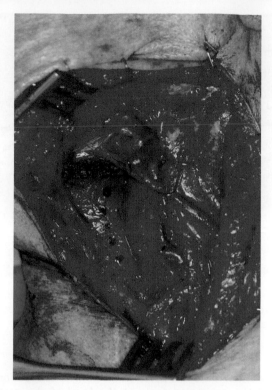

Fig. 25   Cervical esophageal stricture after total laryngectomy. Outline of the proposed release of the stricture.

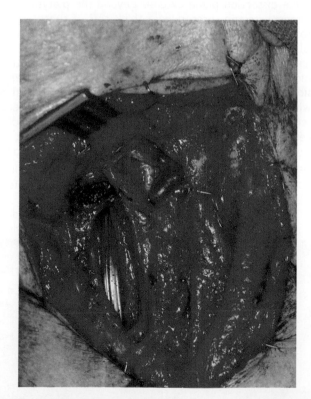

Fig. 26   Relief of the esophageal stricture, showing opening into the cervical esophagus.

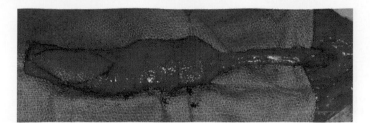

Fig. 27   Harvested RFFF.

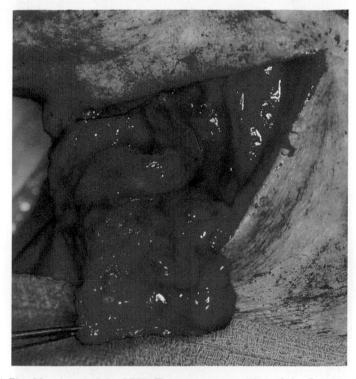

Fig. 28   Inset of the RFFF. The cutaneous portion of the flap was used to reconstruct the esophageal defect.

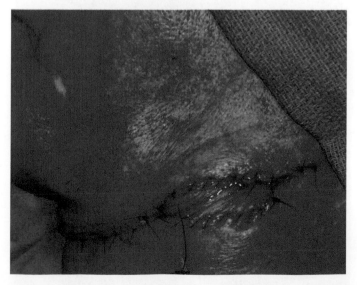

Fig. 29   Closure of cervical wound with external skin paddle for monitoring.

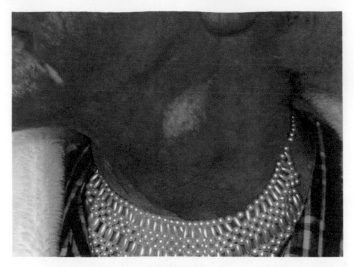

Fig. 30 Follow-up showing healing of the neck wound with no evidence of fistula, and viable flap.

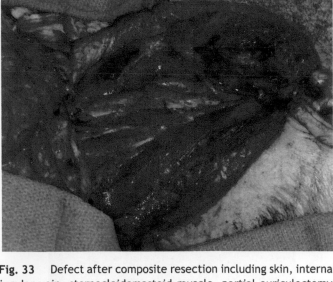

Fig. 33 Defect after composite resection including skin, internal jugular vein, sternocleidomastoid muscle, partial auriculectomy, partial parotidectomy, and neck dissection.

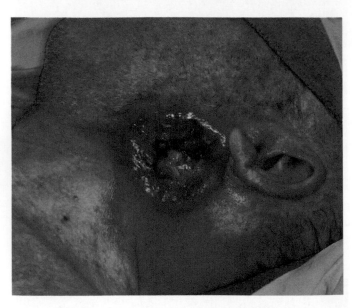

Fig. 31 Large skin cancer left posterior neck.

The incision extends posteriorly from the superiormost aspect of the cervical defect. At the level of the posterior border of the sternocleidomastoid muscle, the incision turns inferiorly and follows the posterior sternocleidomastoid border over the clavicle and into the deltopectoral groove. From there, the incision can be extended below the level of the nipple where it turns medially into the inframammary fold. The last component of the incision should be marked but not incised because it may not be necessary. In the neck, the flap is elevated in the subplatysmal plane. Over the clavicle and chest wall, the dissection plane extends beyond the platysma in a subcutaneous plane, preserving a thick cuff of subcutaneous fat to enhance the viability of the subdermal plexus. The internal mammary perforators are preserved medially as the medial extent of dissection terminates just lateral to their location. The inframammary fold back cut facilitates a considerable degree of cephalad movement of the flap, allowing further rotation of the flap tip into the cutaneous defect if necessary. Flap inset is performed in a standard fashion and the inevitable standing cone is not corrected at the time of initial flap transfer. Standing cone repair is delayed for at least 3 months (Figs. 31–34).

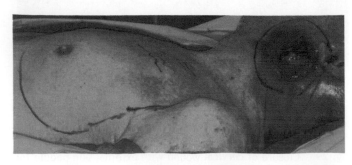

Fig. 32 Outline of planned resection and cervicopectoral flap.

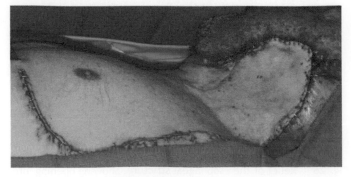

Fig. 34 Closure of the wound with the cervicopectoral flap.

Summary

Reconstruction of various cervical defects can be challenging. Prior oncologic resection combined with radiation therapy compounds the level of difficulty. The judicious application of vascularized flaps, either pedicled or free flaps, can significantly improve the quality of life of cancer survivors with these issues.

References

1. Hui Y, Wei WI, Yuen PW, et al. Primary closure of pharyngeal remnant after total laryngectomy and partial pharyngectomy: how much residual mucosa is sufficient? Laryngoscope 1996;106:490—4.
2. Ariyan S. The pectoralis major myocutaneous flap. A versatile flap for reconstruction in the head and neck. Plast Reconstr Surg 1979; 63(1):73—81.
3. Gendreau-Lefèvre AK, Audet N, Maltais S, et al. Prophylactic pectoralis major muscle flap in prevention of pharyngocutaneous fistula in total laryngectomy after radiotherapy. Head Neck 2014. http://dx.doi.org/10.1002/hed.23742.
4. Gilbert MR, Sturm JJ, Gooding WE, et al. Pectoralis major myofascial onlay and myocutaneous flaps and pharyngocutaneous fistula in salvage laryngectomy. Laryngoscope 2014. http://dx.doi.org/10.1002/lary.24796.
5. Piazza C, Taglietti V, Nicolai P. Reconstructive options after total laryngectomy with subtotal or circumferential hypopharyngectomy and cervical esophagectomy. Curr Opin Otolaryngol Head Neck Surg 2012;20:77—88.
6. Vu KN, Day TA, Gillespie MB, et al. Proximal esophageal stenosis in head and neck cancer patients after total laryngectomy and radiation. ORL J Otorhinolaryngol Relat Spec 2008;70(4):229—35.
7. Di Benedetto G, Aquinati A, Pierangeli M, et al. From the "cherretera" to the supraclavicular fascial island flap: revisitation and further evolution of a controversial flap. Plast Reconstr Surg 2005; 115:70—6.
8. Emerick KS, Herr MA, Deschler DG. Supraclavicular flap reconstruction following total laryngectomy. Laryngoscope 2014;124(8): 1777—82. http://dx.doi.org/10.1002/lary.24530.
9. Yang GF, Chen PJ, Gao YZ, et al. Forearm free skin flap transplantation: a report of 56 cases. 1981. Br J Plast Surg 1997;50(3): 162—5 [Medline].
10. Song YG, Chen GZ, Song YL. The free thigh flap: a new free flap concept based on the septocutaneous artery. Br J Plast Surg 1984; 37:149—59.
11. Welkoborsky HJ, Deichmuller C, Bauer L, et al. Reconstruction of large pharyngeal defects with microvascular free flaps and myocutaneous pedicled flaps. Curr Opin Otolaryngol Head Neck Surg 2013;21:318—27.
12. Seidenberg B, Rosenak S, Hurwitt E, et al. Immediate reconstruction of the cervical esophagus by a revascularized isolated jejunal segment. Am J Surg 1959;149:162—71.
13. Cordova A, D'Arpa S, Di Lorenzo S, et al. Prophylactic chimera anterolateral thigh/vastus lateralis flap: preventing complications in high-risk head and neck reconstruction. J Oral Maxillofac Surg 2014; 72(5):1013—22. http://dx.doi.org/10.1016/j.joms.2013.11.010.

Moving?

Make sure your subscription moves with you!

To notify us of your new address, find your **Clinics Account Number** (located on your mailing label above your name), and contact customer service at:

Email: journalscustomerservice-usa@elsevier.com

800-654-2452 (subscribers in the U.S. & Canada)
314-447-8871 (subscribers outside of the U.S. & Canada)

Fax number: 314-447-8029

Elsevier Health Sciences Division
Subscription Customer Service
3251 Riverport Lane
Maryland Heights, MO 63043

*To ensure uninterrupted delivery of your subscription, please notify us at least 4 weeks in advance of move.

Printed and bound by CPI Group (UK) Ltd, Croydon, CR0 4YY

22/10/2024

01777490-0001